ZAK, MY BOY WONDER

By Joanne Lythgoe and Deb McEwan

The right of Joanne Lythgoe and Deb McEwan to be identified as the authors of this work has been asserted by them in accordance with the Copyright, Designs and Patents Act 1988.

Copyright Joanne Lythgoe and Deb McEwan Cyprus 2019

ISBN: 978-9925-7632-0-7

Note from the authors
Joanne Lythgoe

Hello, I'm Joanne and, first things first, you need to know that I'm a busy mum and businesswoman. I never considered myself to be an author until I talked to my friend, Deb, who is! She's helped me by co-writing this book about my son and my life before, during and after Zak was born. I had many memories safely tucked away in a box until now. But although I've shed lots of tears since deciding to empty that box, the experience has been very cathartic.

This book is a memoir. It reflects my present recollections of experiences garnered over time. I haven't changed any names because most of the people mentioned in this book are friends and family.

Unfortunately, some of the organisations I had to deal with before Zak was born weren't very nice. My memories of these are backed up by sound documentary evidence – if there was one thing Zak's father was really good at, it was keeping records, and I have copies of all the letters to and from the Royal Air Force at that time which corroborates my story, should they be needed in the future.

Deb McEwan

I met Jo and her children when my husband and I moved to Cyprus in 2013. When we got to know each other and she shared her story over a drink one night I was astounded. It's hard to believe that a family could be treated with such cruelty, indifference and a complete lack of compassion and empathy. This sounded like a tale from Victorian times and not the twenty-first century. When I suggested she share her story, she said she was too busy looking after both children – especially Zak who still needed a number of surgeries – and didn't have the emotional or physical energy required to dig up the past. Now that thirteen years have passed since Zak was born, Jo feels ready to share this harrowing but inspirational tale of a woman and her family who refused to give up and were determined not to let the judgemental, nasty, small-minded people* grind them down.

To the people who made the wrong decisions thirteen years ago; I hope karma comes to bite you in the bum.

* (I have resisted using a swear word here as this is a family friendly book.)

Disclaimer

This book is a memoir. It reflects the author's present recollections of experiences over time. Some characteristics have been changed, some events have been compressed, and some dialogue has been recreated.

"Why fit in when you were born to stand out?"

Dr Seuss

Contents

Life Before Zak 11

A Child is Born 22

And Breathe... 37

Leaving Hospital – Reality Hits 64

Down to Business 98

Single Mum 107

The Big Picture 127

From Zak 140

My Boy Wonder 141

Final Thoughts from Jo 143

Life Before Zak

This is the story of my son, Zak Jacob Coates, born against all odds on 24 February 2006. My very own boy wonder...

I met Zak's father, Jake, in Cyprus during the summer of 2005. He was in the Royal Air Force and I worked for a large tour operator as the resort manager. The attraction was instant and Zak was conceived in August 2005, just before my 40th birthday. I don't know about life beginning at forty, but mine changed dramatically that year.

Our family unit was made up of India, my five-year-old daughter from a previous relationship, and Jake's daughters from his first marriage, Lucy (nine) and Hannah (seven). Jake's daughters lived with him and the girls became best friends during their first meeting at Limassol Water Park, when India gave Lucy and Hannah her Barbie dolls to play with.

Prior to meeting Jake, I had been a single mum living

in Cyprus with my five-year-old daughter, India. She had a major health scare when she was a baby; she caught dysentery and failed to recover. We were living in the Dominican Republic at the time and India's health deteriorated rapidly. I worked for a tour operator and was able to take advantage of the first available seats on a flight going to the UK. We flew into Gatwick where my brother-in-law, Glynn, picked us up and drove us straight to Booth Hall Children's Hospital, Manchester. They very quickly put us both into isolation and said that India was suffering from severe malnutrition. Over the course of a week, India was tested for lots of conditions and towards the end of that week she was subjected to an endoscopy procedure where they quickly determined that India had Celiac Disease. Her diet was immediately changed and she began to recover overnight and flourish.

The company I worked for then offered me a job in Cyprus and it was here that this story truly begins.

These were exciting times. We all moved into our new apartment in December 2005 and the only blight on our excitement and happiness was my morning sickness. I'd never experienced anything quite like this, and will never know why it's called morning sickness. For me it was constant throughout the day, and night time too. I looked back on the almost idyllic pregnancy I had with India and was convinced the differences were because I was having a boy. The scan confirmed this. With three girls already in our family we were both delighted with this news and the girls were very excited about having a little brother.

The happiness was short-lived.

Following my twenty-week scan, the sonographer wanted us to return the following week for a second scan.

During that first scan, the sonographer had concentrated on my baby's head. I wracked my brain trying to work out what, if anything could be wrong. Neither Jake nor I knew anything about cleft lips or palates, and we hadn't met anyone with these conditions, but for some reason, I couldn't stop thinking about them. As soon as we arrived home that day I followed my gut instinct and we started researching on the Internet. I was surprised to find that there wasn't much information and most of what we did find came from America. The one UK website that was very useful was the Cleft Lip and Palate Association (CLAPA), the only UK-wide voluntary organisation specifically for anyone affected by cleft lips and palates. I'm still grateful I found this charity as they have been supportive since day one.

During the second scan, I noticed the sonographer was still concentrating on my baby's head. This hadn't happened when I was pregnant with India so the tiny alarm bells that had already been ringing were now loudly clamouring for attention, especially when he told us he was going to get a second opinion. He seemed to take ages checking my baby's head and Jake and I looked at each other. My worries were reflected in his eyes and I was the first to ask the question:

'Are you looking for a cleft?' It was the only question I could think of to ask and to this day, I don't know why.

He seemed surprised that I'd asked that particular question but nodded anyway, agreeing with me that he had noticed something was different. Another doctor came into the room and checked out the scans. He agreed that my baby had some sort of cleft lip, palate or both, but that it was too early to confirm exactly what the problem was. As Jake and I were not married, I was being treated as a private patient. This meant we had to have a discussion about whether our baby would be entitled to medical treatment under the current military rules and regulations. We were assured by one of the midwives that the baby would be covered as a dependant of Jake. We were also informed that because Manchester was my home city, we would be referred to the Manchester Cleft Lip and Palate Team.

At home that evening we looked at some pictures of before and after reconstructive surgery, and reality hit like a bolt of lightning. We had been asked to consider aborting my baby because he was going to have to undergo invasive surgery and suffer dreadfully. My heart bled for this precious bundle I was carrying, and now I understood something of why we had been asked to consider aborting him. However, despite the initial shock, we decided that no matter what happened we already loved him, and we were definitely going to keep our baby whatever challenges lay ahead.

Because I lived overseas, the company I worked for only covered my medical bills for the first part of my pregnancy therefore I was to be relocated back to the UK for the remainder of the pregnancy and maternity leave. Although I was unable to obtain help from the RAF for my own personal treatment, I was allowed to be treated at the military clinic on a private, paying patient, basis. So I chose to stay in Cyprus. As the baby I was carrying was a dependant of Jake's, we were assured he would receive all the medical treatment he needed. The relief of knowing that the baby would be treated was palpable when, following the scan diagnosis, it was determined that our baby would need specialist care when born and the social workers and maternity teams who worked with the military came to my assistance. They ordered special bottles for feeding and connected me with the Manchester Specialist Cleft team.

I was put in touch with Trisha Bannister, a cleft lip and palate coordinator and specialist, who was helpful from the outset. We had numerous conversations where Trisha explained everything from feeding methods (depending on the type of cleft), to the best equipment to be used. It was agreed that at week twenty-eight of my pregnancy I would return to the ante-natal clinic in Cyprus, The Princess Mary Hospital (TPMH), for further scans as they would be able to determine the extent of our baby's cleft. In the meantime, I was advised to discuss any concerns with the coordinator who was more than happy for me to call at any time.

Twenty-five weeks into my pregnancy at an antenatal appointment, it was confirmed that my blood pressure was getting higher and higher. This was the onset of pre-eclampsia. This sometimes life-threatening complication was common in my family. I have two sisters with six children between us, and all of us suffered from pre-eclampsia at various stages of our pregnancies. I had experienced this with India but not until the thirty-ninth week of my pregnancy. My blood pressure rocketed and India's heart rate decreased. Due to the seriousness of the situation the medical team advised an emergency caesarean section, and I agreed. Although small, she was perfectly healthy.

The medical clinic at the Royal Air Force base in Akrotiri prescribed medication to control my blood pressure and advised total rest – as you can imagine this was nigh on impossible with three young girls at home!

To add to an already stressful situation, the midwives

and doctors at the military base now started to question whether our baby *would* be entitled to medical cover after the birth, because we were not married. Their previous assurance that our baby would be entitled to the full-range of medical treatment had influenced our decision to remain in Cyprus for the birth.

Up to this point, we had received all the support we needed under the agreement that any treatment for me was to be paid for by us, but that, as Jake's dependant, the baby would be covered by the military in the same way that other airmen's children were. Jake's two daughters had already had various appointments with doctors in the military system, so we had no reason to believe it would be any different for his son. The military medical authorities had already ordered the specialist feeding bottles (MAM bottles) that our son would need, had put us in touch with the Manchester Cleft Team and on top of that, had given assurances that our baby would be entitled to the full range of medical treatment that he would need. We were more concerned about the seriousness of our baby's cleft than we were about administrative matters.

Oh, how trusting we were!

During the twenty-six-week check-up, my blood pressure was considered abnormally high which was worsened when a female nurse made a passing comment that our son would be 'a bastard'.

On hearing this, I closed my eyes for a second while my brain tried to process what was happening. When I opened them I looked directly at the nurse. I could see nothing about her that suggested to me she would refer to our beloved baby by such a cruel and unkind word and it only added to my stress. Then the locum doctor said that he could give me tranquilizers to enable me to get the first plane home to the UK as soon as possible. He explained that, as I wasn't married to Jake, he couldn't possibly send any medically trained personnel to accompany me, because I was a private patient.

This didn't feel right. 'But wouldn't it be dangerous to give me tranquilizers when I've already got very-high blood pressure and I am 26 weeks pregnant? And there's no medical support on the plane?' I didn't wait for an answer and turned to Jake. 'We need to go to the general hospital now, to see if they will help us.' I felt as if my heart would burst through my chest as I started to panic and wondered what would become of us.

Everything seemed to be happening at once – the doctor carried on suggesting I take certain medication, Jake was understandably upset due to the way they appeared to be withdrawing from our situation, and I was feeling worse by the second. On top of this, they had used an inappropriate and archaic word to describe our unborn child.

I was amazed at the change in attitude of the medical staff, and my panic over the situation meant that my already high blood pressure rocketed. I had been in good health up until this point but got the impression that because my health was deteriorating, the doctors now realised that the treatment was going to cost more than they initially expected, so more statements were made about the fact that Jake and I weren't married, and 'who was entitled to what' raised its ugly head. The military medical authorities decided that now was the time to wash their hands of me, as they knew at this stage I would have to have an emergency caesarean section. However, due to my situation now being considered a medical emergency, the military blue-lighted me to the General Hospital in Nicosia by ambulance, which was approximately seventy kilometres away. The situation was becoming more serious by the minute due to the pre-eclampsia and this was the only place on the island with the appropriate neo-natal facilities and equipment. I was accompanied by a military nurse (a captain) who told me that the military had a duty of care both to me and to our baby. So at this point I started to calm down and to stop worrying; maybe they were going to look after us after all.

Jake was still extremely upset at the way the military and support services had, at this stage, abrogated responsibility. He later spoke to staff at the medical centre and SSAFA – the organisation who employed the midwives and social workers – and was assured that everything would be fine and that, no matter what, they would provide the support needed to look after our baby.

Looking back, I have no idea whether Jake was lied to, or at the very least, intentionally misled.

At the time I had other issues to worry about.

A Child is Born

The nursing care in Makarios III Hospital in Nicosia is completely different to that in the UK. Looking back on my time in the hospital, it felt like the care of pregnant women and new mothers bordered on Victorian. Saying that, their neo-natal ward is the only one in Cyprus and the technology is outstanding.

During a scan I had on arrival at the hospital, it was discovered that our baby had only hours to live if he stayed inside me. This was due both to my ill health and the fact that the placenta was dying – but no care or compassion was shown to Jake or me.

'He's extremely deformed and it would be best if he doesn't survive,' the gynaecologist informed us, very matter-of-factly. This upset and angered both of us, as he didn't understand that we already loved our baby with all our hearts and would do anything in our power to ensure his survival.

Eight hours after arriving at the hospital, following a

number of drugs to try to lower my blood pressure, the decision was made to perform an emergency operation to deliver our baby. At this point, they also administered steroids to help the baby's lungs to develop, prior to him being born. Then they put me on a trolley and, as I was being wheeled into theatre, the surgeon said in a friendly/bright and breezy manner, almost as though he was offering me the choice between a cup of tea or coffee, 'There's only a twenty per cent chance of your baby being born alive, or surviving afterwards.'

As they masked me in theatre and started cutting before I was fully asleep, these words preyed on my mind and my blood ran cold before I lost consciousness.

He was born at 11 am on 24th February 2006, approximately three and a half months early. He weighed a pitiful seven hundred and ninety grams and following an earlier family vote, we named him Zak Jacob Coates.

Whilst I was still unconscious, and immediately after his delivery, Zak was rushed to the neo-natal ward and placed in an incubator. I was in tremendous pain when I eventually came round from the anaesthetic and woke up screaming. There was no morphine drip or continuous pain relief (like there had been when I gave birth to India in the UK). Even so, my eyes searched for Jake's and I uttered the question that was immediately in my head, 'Has our baby died?'

Jake was obviously upset too. 'He's alive,' he said. 'We've had to have him baptized.'

'Why did you do that?' I asked, my heart almost beating out of my chest.

Jake said it was touch and go for our baby and as soon as he was born, the Padre (Armed Forces Chaplain) had advised that Zak should be baptized – in case the worst happened. I struggled to cope with this information, now believing that our baby was at death's door.

'It's okay, his condition is stable now, but still very serious.' Jake tried to reassure me.

Relieved at this news, I was desperate to see Zak, but still in immense pain. Seeing that I was still in agony, Jake asked the nurses for pain relief time and again. He ended up almost begging for it before they gave me an injection to ease the pain. I was then able to think more clearly and it dawned on me that we were entitled to assistance from the Padre, but not from the medics! I was filled with gratitude that the Padre hadn't decided to discriminate against Zak, simply because his parents were not married.

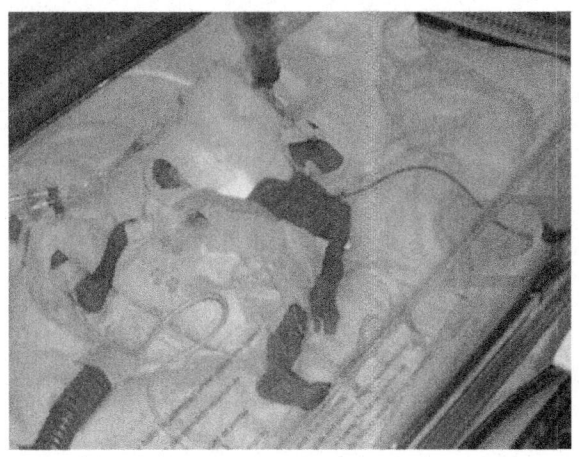

Love at first sight

The first time I set eyes on Zak was the day after he was born, when I was taken down to the NICU in a wheelchair. He was completely covered with wires, and machines were beeping all around him. Although filled with love as I approached Zak's incubator, my other main emotion was fear. Zak was very premature: he was tinier than I expected and the fact that his whole face was bandaged came as a complete shock. The cleft was extreme, but I still thought I'd see Zak's face and was desperate to do so.

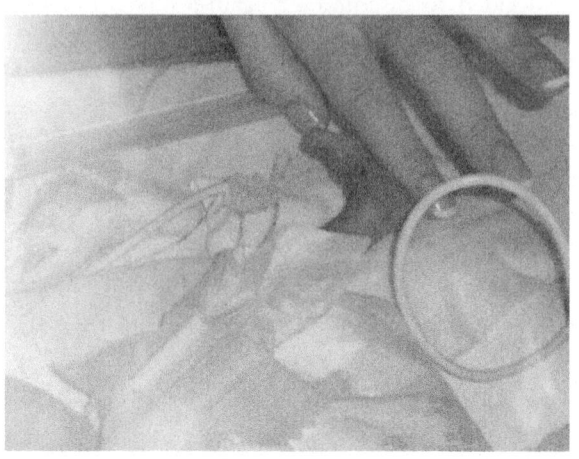

Welcome to the world, Zak

The sound of alarms going off terrified me and I later learnt that this was because Zak's heart rate kept decreasing, and sometimes even stopped. In addition to the tubes and wires, Zak's face was completely covered on the right side, so I had no idea of the extent of his cleft.

The nurses informed me that I couldn't touch Zak and that the doctor wanted to speak to us. I ignored them and placed my hand against the warmth of his tiny foot, desperate for him to know that his mother was there. There wasn't much I could do for my baby, but I could try to express the milk he so desperately needed. Due to the stress I was under, and my general ill health, it took me two days to express one millilitre of liquid. Although it was miniscule, I was very proud of my achievement, but when I tried to give it to the nurse I was sent away like a naughty child, and they refused to give it to him. Maybe at this point the staff already believed my son wouldn't survive.

I fell in love with Zak immediately; an overwhelming love accompanied by the primal desire to protect him. The doctor didn't give us much hope. Not only did Zak have a very severe cleft lip and palate, but his right eye was also affected and he had been born without a lower eyelid or cheekbone. The staff had bandaged over and around his eye and I discovered later that this was the worst thing they could have done as they should have kept his eye lubricated. They admitted that they didn't have the specialist care Zak needed and encouraged us to get him back to the UK as soon as possible.

Following Zak's baptism, Jake was informed by the military that a bed had been made available for him in the neo-natal ward of St James's Hospital in Leeds – famously known as Jimmy's. Once it was determined that he was stable enough to fly, Zak would be casevaced (a term the military use when they airlift a wounded person to a place where he can be treated in safety) by air ambulance and I was to accompany him.

While all this was happening, I was so glad to see my sister, Melanie, and Jake's mother, Dorothy, who had both travelled to Cyprus as soon as they knew I'd been rushed into hospital. They were a wonderful source of comfort in those early days both for Jake and I, and although Ashra – our full-time nanny - was looking after the girls at home, Dorothy and Melanie were a great help.

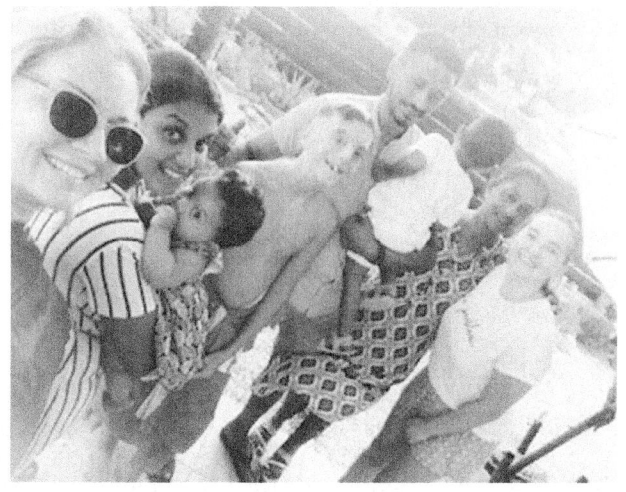

A recent photo of Ashra and her family with me, India, and Zak

Two days later I was in bed and Jake was at my side when Karen, a nurse I'd met before (rank of captain), arrived from the military base. She took a seat on a chair at the right-hand side of my bed, and was armed with an official looking clipboard, and pen and paper. She started to fidget, which made me think she was uncomfortable and was likely to impart news that we didn't want to hear.

'Questions are being asked,' she said, before informing us that the air ambulance had been cancelled due to Zak being 'non-entitled.'

'Because you're not married, there is no obligation to look after your son.'

We were devastated.

'What do you mean?' I asked and looked at Jake. I was new to the military way of life but my partner was in the Royal Air Force. Had she really told me that they had no responsibility to help us and to look after our son, just because Jake and I weren't married? Was this really the attitude of the British Forces in the twenty-first century?

I couldn't get my head around what she was saying. 'You do know that Jake is divorced and that his daughters are already entitled to the same benefits as other children whose fathers are in the RAF?' I asked.

Jake was as shocked, angry, and upset as I was. He asked many questions but the answers were always the same.

'I can go back and ask,' she said. 'But the air ambulance is cancelled and the bed in St James's too. Sorry, but our only responsibility is to the father and not to the baby.'

This was despite all the reassurances that Jake had received, so my earlier optimism had been in vain.

Jake had served for over twenty-four years in the Royal Air Force, including a stint on operations, yet his son was not entitled to medical treatment from the forces simply because his parents weren't married. We were informed that the British High Commission would be asked to assist us. I have obtained a copy of the email sent by Personnel/Welfare at Headquarters British Forces Cyprus to the British High Commission and I quote:

'The Chain-of-command at British Forces Cyprus will not accept responsibility for mother and child due to illegitimate birth mother and father not married. British Forces Cyprus accept responsibility for father only.

No birth certificate has been applied for. Again, birth certificate will not be issued by British Forces Cyprus due to illegitimate birth.'

The only organisation within the forces community that showed us any care or compassion were SSAFA, (the oldest military charity to whom the MOD contract to provide secondary healthcare and social services in Cyprus), some of whom were flabbergasted that we were being treated in this way. We were both devastated on discovering the Royal Air Force had abandoned any duty of care towards one of its own, his partner, and their very sick baby. Had we been informed of this earlier in my pregnancy and had Jake not been given false reassurance, I would have returned to the UK to give birth, as I had with India. The British High Commission explained that they would help us with the paperwork we needed to travel and organise the air ambulance, but we would have to pay for the flight at a cost of approximately £100,000.00 There was no need for me to check our bank accounts to know that we didn't have that sort of money. The British High Commission were very sympathetic and also couldn't understand why the Royal Air Force were treating us in this way.

The hospital was still adamant that we needed to get Zak to the UK for specialist treatment as soon as possible, especially for his eye.

While all this was going on, I was still being monitored by the hospital for my high blood pressure, due to the severe pre-eclampsia I had suffered. My stress levels and hormones were all over the place, worsened by the abandonment of us by the Royal Air Force. I wasn't in a very good place at all but knew I had to overcome this because my baby boy needed all my love and attention.

To put things into perspective, military personnel and their families stationed at Royal Air Force Akrotiri in Cyprus receive medical treatment and any other support on a par with what they can expect to receive in the UK. I wasn't aware that being unmarried would affect the treatment received for our baby – or perhaps I should say lack of treatment. They washed their hands of us completely and we even had to sort out an emergency passport and birth certificate for Zak; a task normally provided by the British Military authorities who would arrange the issue of a British Birth Certificate. Although the British High Commission helped with this, it was still traumatic having to travel around Nicosia to find a court that could provide all of the certificates I needed to be able to get the documents, while worrying about my very seriously ill, new-born baby, and recovering from major surgery. In the end, we were issued with a Cypriot Birth Certificate when our son was fully entitled to a British document. Again, this was all done without any help or support from the Royal Air Force.

During my stay in the hospital I met another new mother in a similar situation. Helen was also a single mum and had been rushed into the hospital when she went into premature labour. Her son, David, was put into intensive care and Helen was only allowed to see him for an hour each day. We took some comfort from each other in those first few days, but lost touch after leaving the hospital.

By now I was at the end of my tether with stress and worry over Zak, but it was at this point I discovered a small light at the end of the tunnel.

I briefly mentioned my company's health insurance policy earlier. Well, I re-read it and realised that I was covered for any medical complications in my pregnancy up to twenty-seven weeks. Zak had been born at twenty-six weeks and four days. My company insurance agreed to help us and they were excellent. Everything was sorted out within seven days and Zak was deemed stable enough to travel to the UK by air ambulance, albeit still in his incubator.

It was decided that I was well enough to be discharged from hospital when Zak was five days old, although it was going to take another week before we were to be air ambulanced to the UK.

I had not been given any bills for my medical treatment so far, so the question of money hadn't arisen, and it was low on my list of priorities as my mind was constantly occupied with worry over the health of our baby. However, as I prepared to leave the hospital the RAF heaped a final indignity onto my head; I was handed a bill for £4500 Cypriot pounds and told that the Royal Air Force representative had informed the hospital to '*Bill Miss Lythgoe.*'

The anger and upset I felt towards the Royal Air Force was considerable. Not only had Zak been born extremely prematurely and was seriously ill due to that fact, he also had a very severe form of cleft lip and palate, and was now blind in one eye. As the hospital staff had had no idea what to do about Zak's eye and had kept it covered, a cyst/scar tissue had developed and this would eventually lead him to lose all sight in that eye. I still hold the Royal Air

Force responsible for Zak's blindness – a situation I now know could have been avoided had he received the correct and timely treatment.

And Breathe...

Leaving the hospital with Zak on 10th March 2006 was very emotional. I was returning to the UK with Zak but had to leave the rest of my family in Cyprus. Because of the language barrier and the complex care needed for my baby, I felt we would both be better off in a hospital in the UK, and close to members of my family.

I needed a routine for the girls who still had to go to school, and yet again, the Royal Air Force continued to make our lives more difficult than they should have been. This time, they were undecided on whether to give Jake compassionate leave while I was away due to my status in his life, and that of our baby. This was like pouring salt on an open wound and I felt like we were being victimised just because we didn't have a marriage certificate.

The travel process involved an English doctor and nurse who would accompany me in the ambulance to the hospital in Nicosia then transfer Zak from his hospital incubator to the travel incubator. Watching all the wires and tubes being taken out of my tiny baby and then others being put back into him, was very traumatic in itself. Once the ambulance departed for Larnaca airport, Jake and I followed by car and we were directed straight onto the tarmac. I watched the medics transfer Zak in his incubator onto the Learjet and, after a hasty goodbye to Jake, I got onto the plane and we took off straight away. On board, there was only the pilot, the doctor and nurse who had been in the ambulance with us, and me and Zak. I was only allowed to take a small suitcase and I had no idea when I'd return to Cyprus, or whether my son would see this Mediterranean island ever again.

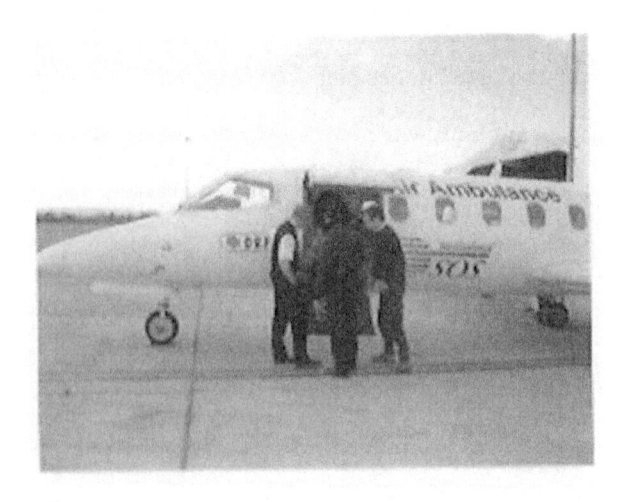

Our air ambulance

After a quick stopover in Baden Baden, Germany, we took off again and headed for Manchester airport.

The doctor and nurse talked about Zak with me during the flight. They explained that although his ventilation was very high, his condition was stable. This was a relief and none of the machines Zak was wired up to bleeped a warning during the entire flight. I still hadn't seen my baby's face, but I slowly started to feel better. Whether this was because I was able to discuss the situation with medical staff who shared the same culture and outlook as I did, or because they had shown me some consideration and compassion, I'm not sure. What I am sure of is that for the first time since Zak's birth, I began to feel cautiously optimistic.

On arrival at Manchester airport in the UK, we transferred to the Manchester Children's Hospital, Neo-Natal Ward. I'm glad I didn't know at the time that this was to be our home for the next four months.

The ambulance from St Mary's Hospital met us on the tarmac, transferred the incubator and took us straight to the hospital. This time I travelled in the ambulance with my son.

We arrived at the hospital in the middle of the night and the reverse process was followed regarding Zak and his incubator. The large team of medical personnel there to greet us were also concerned about my feelings and health. One of the receiving nurses put an arm around me and this small act of compassion opened the floodgates. From arrival I was spoken to and told what was happening during every step of the way. As well as the wonderfully overwhelming greeting, I was a twenty-minute drive from my family – my Mum and my sisters, Melanie, Shelley, and their families.

Once I'd composed myself, I was asked to give the nurses my milk. They were shocked when I explained that I didn't have any, as I had been told in Cyprus that they would not feed my milk to Zak.

Zak was taken to the NICU (Neo-Natal Intensive Care Unit) and, once settled, I was shown to the room I would be staying in. A nurse provided a machine so I could express my milk and I was asked to get to work straight away.

This soon became an obsession and, as well as the NICU freezer containing vast amounts of my expressed milk, my sister had to remove everything from her freezer at home to accommodate numerous bottles of milk for Zak. For months after, wherever I went, my milk machine came with me

I was informed that the next few months would be a major rollercoaster ride – and how true that turned out to be! After arrival in intensive care, Zak was immediately removed from the travel incubator and his care was taken over by a multitude of doctors and nurses. It was both refreshing and reassuring to actually be spoken to by a member of Zak's medical team. In Cyprus, we had to make arrangements to speak to the doctor between one and two pm, and even then we had to join a queue outside his door which made us feel like naughty children waiting outside the headmaster's office for our punishments.

Once I knew Zak was in safe hands, I fell asleep, exhausted. When I awoke a few hours later, I immediately went to check on him. The nurses were so kind and caring that it made me cry – as you will discover, I cried a lot during those first few weeks – but the tears were also those of relief, knowing that Zak would now have the excellent medical care that he so needed and deserved.

The day after our arrival at the hospital, a number of family members came to visit, and so did a large number of specialist staff. When I look back on this day now, I realise it passed in a complete blur, but the major memory I have is of the relief I felt at being back in the bosom of my extended family, knowing that, whatever happened, they would be there to support me together with the talented, caring, and compassionate medical staff. This was also the day when a name was put to Zak's cleft: it was a Tessier Type 4 Bilateral Cleft Lip and Palate affecting the right side of his face, including his eye. This is an extremely rare condition with less than fifty cases reported worldwide.

When I saw Zak that morning, everything had changed. His bandages had been removed and I saw the extent of his cleft for the first time. Although I had carried out a lot of research on babies born with clefts, nothing had prepared me for the extent of my baby's cleft. It was a shock because the cleft was far more complex than I could ever have imagined and because it also affected his eye. During my research I had never seen a Tessier Cleft. Once his condition had a name, I Googled to find more information but it was very limited due to the rarity of the condition.

Love and a fierce surge of protection welled through me, and I vowed to do whatever it took to help my baby boy as much as I could.

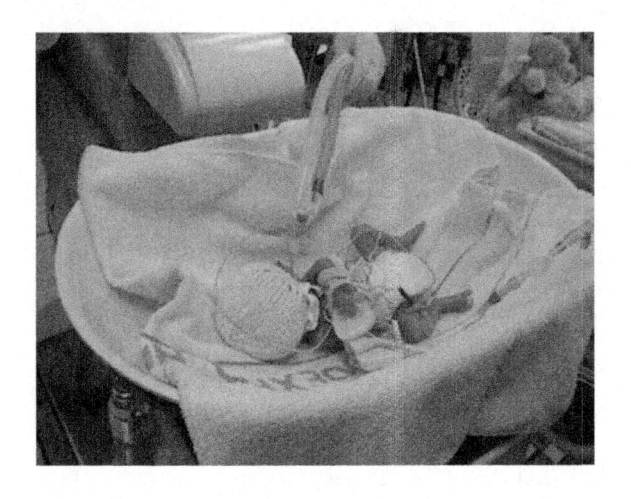

The first weigh-in

This was also the first opportunity I had to hold Zak. When the staff told me what was to happen, I misread the signals. Fear hit me like a bolt of lightning; I thought they wanted me to hold my baby so that I could say goodbye to him.

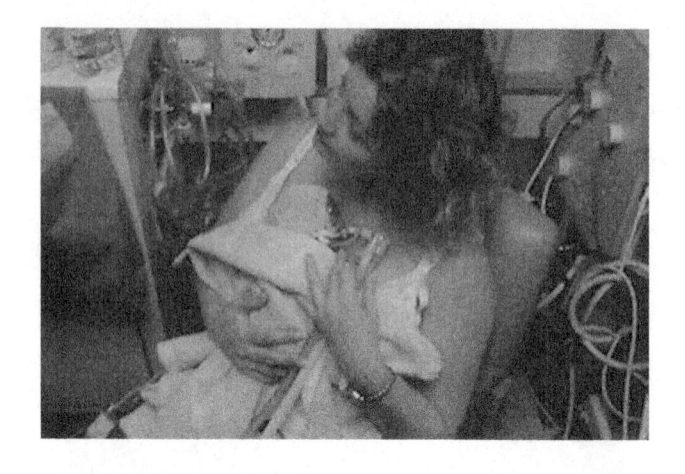

Kangaroo care – the first time I held my precious baby

Still highly ventilated, with all the wires attached, Zak was put down my bra and we had skin-to-skin contact (known as kangaroo care) for two hours. In those two hours his saturations (blood pressure/stability etc) were the best they had ever been. I was overwhelmed with emotion when I realised that encouraging mothers to have more input and contact with their baby was a normal occurrence in a British NICU. I didn't move and spent the time revelling in the smell and feel of my precious boy.

Holding Zak was absolute bliss and I didn't want to put him back in his box!

*****

I had a long conversation with the doctors shortly after arrival at St Mary's Hospital, and was shocked and horrified by some of the information given to me:

- Zak had been given numerous blood transfusions in hospital in Cyprus.
- He had a number of blood clots on his brain.
- He had a small valve opening in his heart.
- He was on the maximum ventilation, possibly due to the fact that his lungs were so under-developed he could not breathe on his own.
- His right eye had developed a cyst/scar tissue due to lack of lubrication whilst in hospital in Cyprus. The implication of this was not made clear to us (while in Cyprus) and I do believe the hospital in Cyprus were unaware of the consequences. However, I now discovered that, due to the scar, Zak's eye could not develop properly and he is now blind in that eye. For those who don't already know, babies are born blind. When they open and close their eyes the

optic nerve reacts and kicks in. Because Zak's eye was covered, this natural process didn't happen, and as he did not have a bottom eyelid, he was unable to blink and his eye dried up. This caused the cyst/scar tissue to form over it to help to protect the eye. The Ocular Plastics Team explained that whilst the scar tissue should remain to protect Zak's eye, his sight had already been compromised and he was therefore most certainly blind in his right eye. However, he is able to distinguish between light and dark from this eye, so there may be hope that Zak can gain some sight in this eye in the future. This will not be determined until Zak's full reconstruction surgery is completed on his bottom eyelid, which will be by the time Zak is seventeen years old.

- He had jaundice.
- He had chromosome tests to check for any syndromes. The genetics specialist in Manchester explained that some babies with certain syndromes also have clefts.
- Zak had been given supplements to keep him

alive, but had not been given any milk.

- His weight at birth was 790 grams and on arrival in Manchester at two weeks old he weighed 700 grams (1.54 pounds).

Within our first week in Manchester many doctors and specialists visited us. In particular, the day after our arrival, four specialists from the Ocular Plastics Team came to examine Zak. They wanted to treat him as a matter of urgency to try to save his eye. They returned a day later with special sutures to try to close Zak's upper eyelid – a temporary fix to protect his eye. A surgery plan was arranged. They wanted his eye to be able to lubricate itself but he would initially need help with this so they prescribed lubrications to be administered daily. It was at this point that I became more involved with Zak's daily care routine, changing nappies, cleaning, and lubricating his eye. Being more involved was very empowering and I now felt more like Zak's mum rather than a spectator in the drama that was my son's life. Although I was allowed to stay with Zak for as long as I wanted and to help as much as I could, the only downside was that I soon became obsessed with the ventilator and the many monitors which were constantly bleeping.

Maybe this is understandable because they were keeping Zak alive - if there wasn't any noise, I knew my baby's life was in jeopardy.

After a few weeks, the specialist teams got together and wrote a plan for Zak's future treatment. I was invited into the NICU Senior Consultant's Office, together with the Plastic Surgeon and a member of the Cleft Team. It was explained to me that they would work in conjunction with each other to do everything they could for Zak, and the plan went right up until he reached the age of seventeen. However, Zak was still on full ventilation and his condition was very serious. Every time the doctors tried to reduce his ventilation he stopped breathing, known as apnea, causing bradycardia (a drop in his blood oxygen level), and he struggled to breathe because his lungs were so weak. As he became stronger and started to grow and his organs developed, they continued to try to reduce the ventilation. His condition was constantly up and down and I felt like I was on a massive rollercoaster ride. I remember one occasion, when Zak was having a few bad days, a nurse screened another incubator and there was a lot of activity around that area. I, and the other parents, were asked to leave. When I returned to the ward later, the screened incubator was missing. It hit home just how serious our situation was, and although Zak's care was superb, he still had a long way to go.

Round about this time I was concerned that Zak wouldn't have any eyelashes! I don't know why this became an obsession with everything else that was going on, but I'm relieved to say that his eyelashes did start to grow so I could concentrate on the bigger picture. Isn't it funny how the mind works in times of crisis?

Nearing the first Mother's Day towards the end of March, India and her sisters were on my mind. The nurses said I could do with a break and I wondered whether I should return to Cyprus. My emotions were in turmoil because I didn't want to leave Zak, but I was well aware that I had other parental responsibilities and I missed them so much, especially India. Zak's condition was still serious but he was stable and the nurses encouraged me to go for a few days (I think they wanted some space in their freezer as well!).

Nicola, one of the wonderful NICU Nurses, gave me this beautiful card before I left, which I treasure to this day.

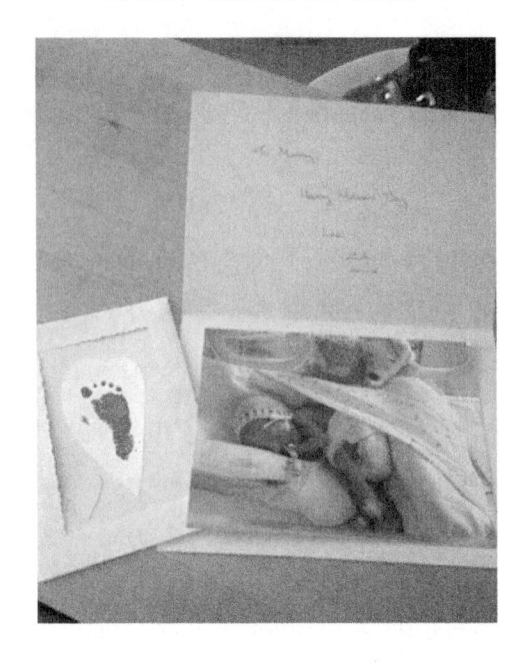

My beautiful Mother's Day card from Nicola

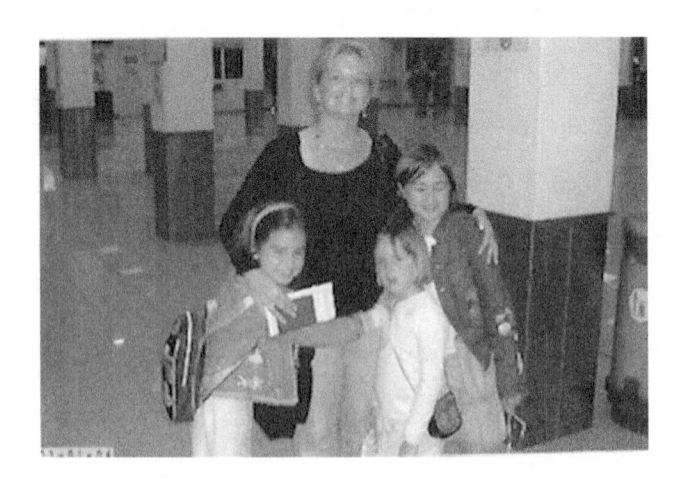

Reunited with the girls

So I flew home. Although it was it lovely to be there and to see my family, Zak was constantly on my mind. My close friends, Liz and Jennie, insisted on a night out. I cried from the time I met them until the time I returned home. During this outing we went for dinner and also visited a club. I ended up feeling so much better for it but I attracted many funny looks and sympathy. People approached Liz and Jennie to ask if I was okay as they couldn't ask me directly because I was sobbing uncontrollably. Looking back, we can all laugh about this now.

During the school holidays, Jake and the girls came over to visit a few times. The first time Jake held him, Zak stopped breathing and turned blue. His heart slowed to almost a stop and a nurse had to resuscitate him while he was in Jake's arms. This was very scary for Jake who hadn't personally experienced how ill Zak was.

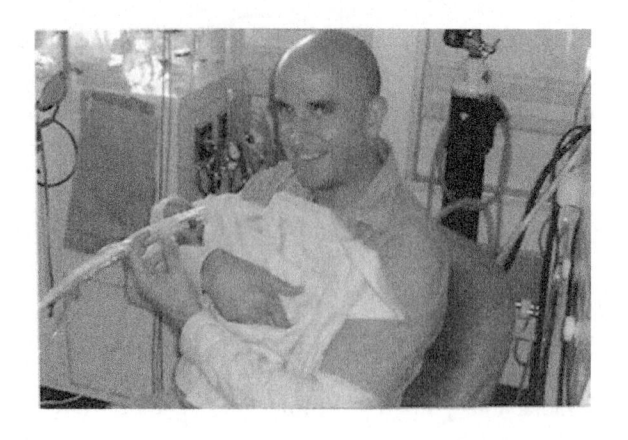

Jake holding Zak for the first time

While all this was going on, my mum was recovering from a stroke. We discovered later that a brain tumour had caused her stroke but whether mum knew about the tumour and decided not to tell us, or was unaware of it herself, we'll never know.

Her health started to deteriorate rapidly and she became a patient in Christie's Hospital, and then I had to coordinate visits between both my mum and my son. When she came to visit Zak, he was in Room 1 of the Intensive Care Unit. She wasn't herself because the brain tumour was growing by the day but I think she knew Zak was her grandson, although it is hard to say for definite. I'm so glad that they did meet each other, as my mother's health went downhill very quickly after this.

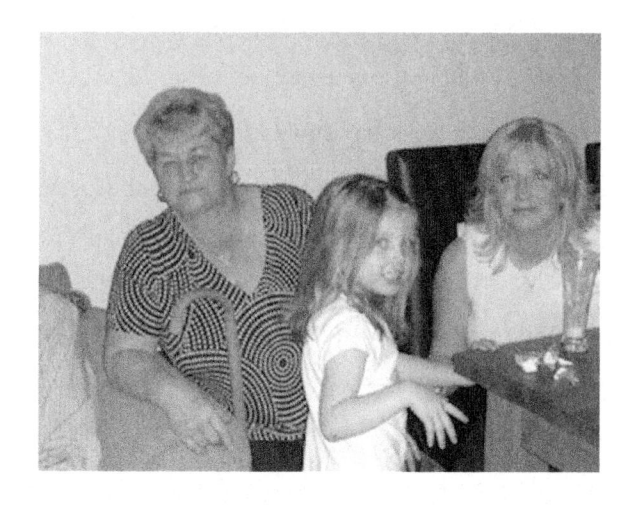

Mum at her sixtieth birthday party, with my sister, Melanie and niece, Hope

After about two and a half months of trying, the staff managed to lower Zak's ventilation levels and we then had talks about Zak's future care. He was in the NICU Room 1 because he was still fully ventilated – once babies are moved to Room 2 you begin to realise there may be light at the end of the tunnel. During our conversations, I was informed that Zak could not be put onto a CPAP (Continuous Positive Airway Pressure) machine for respiratory support (which is generally the second step with premature babies to wean them off oxygen support), as the anatomy of his face would not allow this because it was too open. Zak did not have a fully formed nose so the machine could not be attached. The staff suggested that a Perspex box could be placed over Zak's head – like a big bubble – for them to deliver ambient oxygen.

This happened when Zak was almost three months old and, unbeknownst to me, was planned for when I wasn't at the hospital. The staff knew how distressing it could be for me to see the tubes and wires being taken away from Zak, so I think this was intentional, and it was the right decision because when I came to visit later that day, I did panic. When I walked into Room 1 and Zak wasn't in his incubator, I thought the worst. His incubator was at the far left window of the room, with a view to Manchester City Football Ground and the whole skyline. This had been our home and view for four months. We had personalised Zak's incubator with our own blankets, photographs and cuddly toys, and the incubator now there, wasn't his. I quickly looked around and Zak's incubator was missing. It was only a few seconds but I think one of the nurses must have seen the expression of horror on my face. She rushed towards me, accompanied by two other nurses. When I saw their big smiles, I realised that all was well.

'Come on,' one of them said. 'We have someone to show you.'

I followed them to Room 2 (the Special Care Room) where Zak lay in his incubator with his little bubble over his head. It was the first time I had seen my baby without all his tubes and he was beautiful. I burst into tears again at this point, and thought I'd never stop. Maybe, just maybe, he might actually live and flourish.

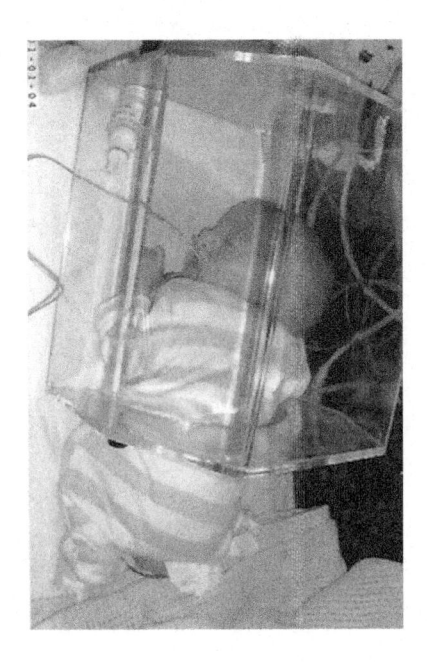

Zak in his 'bubble'

Later that day I was allowed to bathe and dress him. In Room 1 (the Intensive Care Room) babies are not dressed, mainly because it's easier for the medical staff to see the babies' chest movements and to judge how well they are. It's also extremely difficult to dress your baby with all the wires and monitors attached.

This was about the same time that Jake told me he had submitted a formal complaint to his chain of command in the Royal Air Force, about their dreadful treatment and lack of compassion. We were both still very upset about this but I had to put it out of my mind so that I could concentrate on my number one priority; Zak's health and wellbeing.

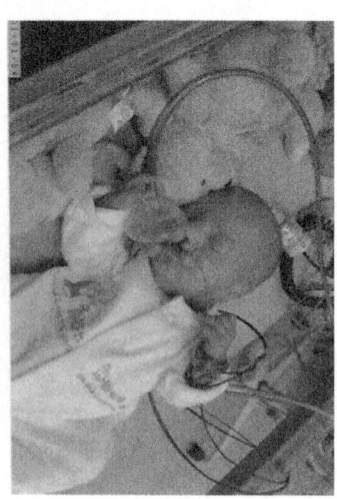

Zak taking ambient oxygen

Zak remained stable and took the ambient oxygen for quite a few days. Eventually, the Perspex bubble was removed and low levels of ambient oxygen were circulated throughout the incubator. I was excited when they told me that Zak could now be removed from it for short periods of time. An oxygen hose was placed near his chest to assist with his breathing and heart rate monitors were also attached. I was allowed to bathe my baby for the first time when he was three months old and it took three of us to do it, due to the wires and other equipment. This was about a week before Zak's due date had my pregnancy reached full-term.

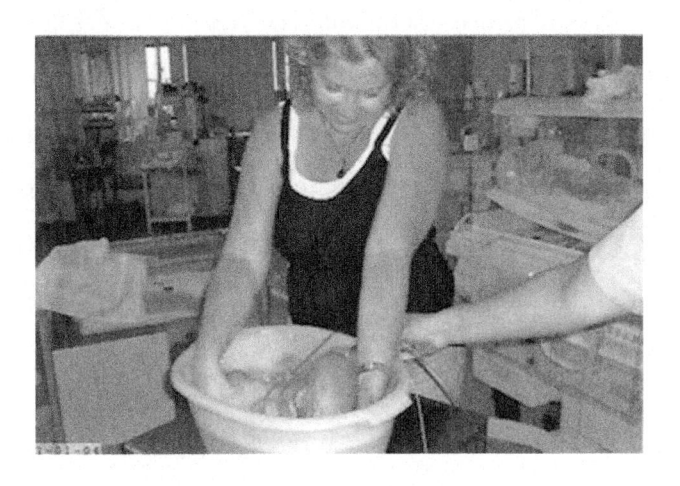

Bathing my beautiful baby for the first time

Zak's condition continued to improve on an almost daily basis and I began to feel like a normal mum. I could now administer his daily care needs, such as changing him, bathing and dressing him, and his dependence on additional oxygen was becoming less and less. Zak was ready to move to Room 3 (Rehab and preparation to leave hospital) when no additional oxygen was needed. Once we had moved I was able to take Zak outside in a pram. I brought his new pram into the hospital and a short outing into the fresh air involved planning and preparation akin to a military operation! I was accompanied by two nurses who had loaded the pram with oxygen bottles, masks and monitors, just in case Zak had a setback and needed to be resuscitated. Imagine a family getting ready for a road trip with the luggage packed around the kids, and multiply that by fifty! The plan was to go out for thirty minutes around the park near to the city's universities, and I was so excited that I didn't sleep properly the night before.

However, quite soon after leaving the hospital front entrance, my spirit was dampened. We crossed the road en route to the park and a woman approached. She asked if I had a new baby, obviously curious because I was with two nurses – my very own bodyguards. She looked in the pram and recoiled; obviously shocked at seeing the extent of Zak's cleft. It was like a punch to my stomach and my very first taste of what was to come. I knew then that I'd turn into Mama Bear and do anything to protect my young cub. My proud mummy moment was now completely shattered and the optimism I'd felt on leaving the hospital quickly turned to worry. I couldn't stop thinking about what Zak would have to go through every time somebody looked at him. My hormones went into overdrive and the love I felt for my son was accompanied by an almost fierce urge to protect him from anyone and everyone. At this point I could have quite easily locked both of us into a room and remained in isolation for ever - not to hide Zak from the world, to me he was the most beautiful boy ever, but to protect him from the stares and comments I knew his unique looks would attract.

Despite Zak's incredible improvements, all was not roses. He struggled to take a full bottle and had to be supplemented with tube feeds known as NG tubes. With cleft feeding bottles, the feeder has to sync to the baby's sucking motion. There is a certain knack to this and it can be very frustrating if you can't get the hang of it. Cleft babies take in a lot of air whilst feeding and the milk can come back out of their nose, as well as their mouths. Babies use a natural reflex action involving sucking, breathing and swallowing to feed and forming a vacuum is what allows them to suck. Some babies with a cleft aren't able to form this vacuum because of the gap in their lip and/or palate, so feeding from a regular bottle or a breast is extremely difficult.

Before he was discharged I had to be taught how to tube feed properly, and I had lessons for this over a period of at least two weeks. This was vitally important because if the tube was placed incorrectly, Zak could have had breathing problems, pneumonia and cardiac or respiratory arrest. I also had to be alone with Zak for a full night to prove I could deal with any problems that might arise. The NICU deal with this by having mother and baby rooms attached to the ward where you are left to your own devices, but know you can call for help if needed. This gives mothers of previously seriously ill babies the confidence to know they can look after their children and, having been in the hospital for almost four months with trained staff and monitors to attend to all of your baby's needs, the first night alone with the baby is very disconcerting. Zak was off all of his monitors at this stage and this was his chance to prove he was ready to start life outside the hospital walls. For most of the night I sat up in bed reading, and drinking coffee. Fear and apprehension meant I didn't get a wink of sleep as I was up and down all night, constantly checking that he was breathing. Zak took his tube feeds and had a peaceful night. In fact, he slept... like a baby!

Discharge day came soon after and it was almost like the first few days after your baby is born and you're taking them home from hospital. Except it wasn't and I was terrified.

I was torn between wanting to take him home to start a relatively normal life, and wanting to stay within the security of the hospital.

All the medical staff were fabulous and I cannot stress enough how supportive they all were, not only for Zak but also for me and my family. I especially remember the NICU nurses because I was closest to them. There was one-on-one care from the nurses who I consider to be very special ladies who helped me, as well as Zak, to get through this very traumatic period.

I formed a friendship with one in particular. Her name was Nicola McCormick and she was one of Zak's NICU nurses. She was the lady who sent me photos of Zak when I had a weekend away from the hospital, to reassure me that everything was going well, and gave me that wonderful Mother's Day card. Sadly, Nicola is no longer with us but I've recently been in touch with her mother. She remembers Zak, and Nicola used to share stories with her mum about Zak's progress. Words can't express how much Nicola's help and care meant to me at the time and I'll never forget her.

Rest in Peace, Nicola, I know you're an angel now.

The hospital had been my second home for the whole period and I was both sad and apprehensive to be leaving. Zak had received twenty-four-hour care for all of his life so far and now I was to be his sole carer. I was used to him having his heart monitor on and the thought that I could not take it home with me completely freaked me out.

We left the hospital on 24th June with me knowing this wasn't to be the end of Zak's visits and treatments. He was to remain under the special care team until he turned two, and would require regular check-ups with the Cleft Team and Occular Plastics, indefinitely.

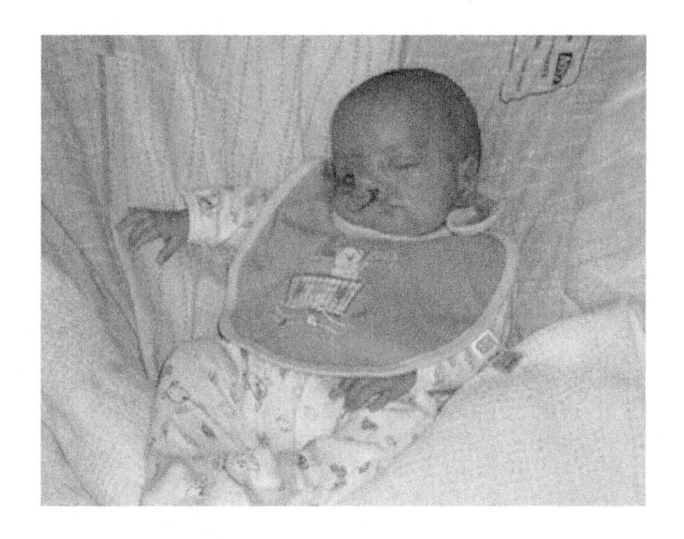

The day we left hospital – I was so nervous

Leaving Hospital – Reality Hits

Though part of me wanted to leave the hospital, it was like cutting the umbilical cord and I would have been happy to take a nurse home with me. We had been in Room 3 for a few weeks where there was still twenty-four hours a day care, but they rehabilitate patients and families to prepare them for life outside the hospital. The obvious way forward was for Zak to live as normal a life as possible. However, he did still have a feeding tube, which I had been trained to use and to change. It was great that he was well enough for this to happen but after almost four months of twenty-four hours a day support I was nervous and anxious, as well as very excited. My sister, Melanie, picked us up and we stayed with her and her family who were very excited to see us. We took over my niece Robyn's room, and turned the house upside down within one hour of arriving. This was to become the routine during future visits for many years to come.

That first week was a whirlwind of activity. The Cleft Team, Health Visitors, Midwives, and the Community Children's Nurse (CCN) came to check on Zak as well as friends and extended family members. The CCN wanted to check that Zak's tube feeding was going to plan. The feeding tube is inserted and can be left in or taken out after every feed. It went through Zak's (very open) nose and down the back of his throat, down the oesophagus (swallowing tube) and directly into his tummy. The tube is made of a thin soft plastic and was taped to the side of Zak's face to keep it secure. The most stressful and difficult aspect of the whole process was ensuring that I placed the tube correctly. It was fiddly and I didn't want to cause Zak any more discomfort than I had to. He was so good when I was doing this. Once the tube was in place I had to attach a syringe with his milk in and just place it higher than Zak. Gravity then takes over and the milk gently flowed into his tummy. During this period, I also persevered with the cleft bottles. The paraphernalia and supplies that came with this was unbelievable – tubes/syringes/fixing tape etc., yet more stuff to clutter up Melanie's house!

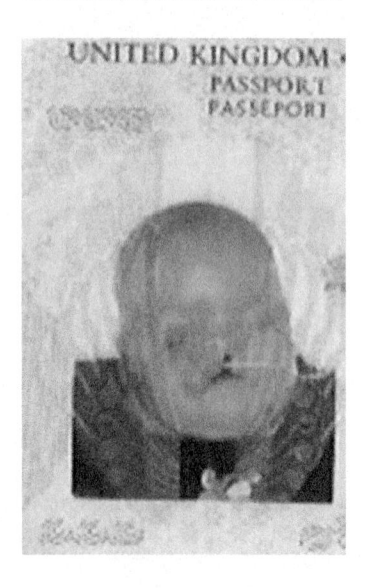

Zak's passport photo shows his feeding tube

As I mentioned, I had been trained to do this, but it was still very stressful. I had been doing this for a week in the hospital without any issues as well as trying to get Zak to take milk from his special bottles. On one occasion when we were at Melanie's home, I put the tube in and discovered it was incorrectly placed when Zak started to gag, and his lips turned blue. This frightened me so badly, I removed the tube immediately! Thankfully Zak began to take to his bottles and I was able to continue feeding him this way, closely monitoring his weight, which increased, meaning he was thriving. After the scare I had when Zak gagged on his tube, and although these were the specialised feeding bottles and Zak's palate was completely open, it was better than using the tube. Possibly pre-empting the problem I had, the hospital had also thoughtfully taught me how to use the bottles properly. From this point Zak went from strength to strength.

Melanie, her husband Glynn, and my nieces, Robyn and Hope, were extremely patient and supportive. They never complained about us or all the equipment we needed for Zak - not to mention taking up their entire freezer with the milk I expressed for Zak. After not being allowed to give Zak my own milk whilst I was in Cyprus, expressing it was still an obsession with me. While in the hospital, I became very competitive, having an overwhelming need to produce more than any other new mother.

'We'll be able to start our own dairy if you carry on like this,' said a nurse, chuckling at the look of utter perplexity that must have been written all over my face.

'Why?' I asked.

'Because all our freezers are filled to overflowing!'

I laughed along with her, but I had no intentions of slowing down. My son needed to be fed, and I was the woman to do it! At one point I was asked to slow down and produce less due to the surplus amount in the freezers. This didn't change when we left hospital and I could have supplied a number of supermarkets. I believe this was born of the desire to do as much as I could as Zak's mother. There wasn't much I could do for him when he was seriously ill in hospital so this helped to satisfy my maternal instincts and also fed my competitive nature. In hindsight, it is obvious that my obsessive desire to feed my son was born from not being able to do much for him when he had been so seriously ill.

We stayed at Mel and Glynn's for a few weeks. During this time, we had lots of hospital appointments and were monitored by the extended team of helpers. I also applied for Zak's new passport.

The medical staff were happy that I could manage Zak on my own and I had a hankering to return to my family in Cyprus. I spoke to a NICU nurse about this shortly after.

'Would Zak be able to fly or is it too soon?' I asked,

even though Zak was thriving and didn't need any additional oxygen. I was fearful that if something were to happen on the plane, there wouldn't be the medical support we needed.

I was told there would always be a risk, but the consensus of all the professionals was, 'He can fly and will be okay.'

So a decision was made that we could go home to Cyprus for a few months, but would return to the hospital for Zak's first surgery on his palate, in September. This was to be the second flight of Zak's short life so far, and I was nervous. It was stressful trying to manage Zak, his feeding equipment and luggage. The thought of getting on a flight with him but without any medical assistance scared me (for reasons stated before), but I had been assured that all would be well, and it was.

I contacted the airline and explained the situation. I had to have extra luggage that a parent with a premature baby would have – extra bottles, premature baby special milk (even though I was expressing, I couldn't keep my milk fresh). Calpol supplies, extra dummies, extra blankets, extra nappies, everything but the kitchen sink! Melanie and Glynn dropped us at the airport and I remember them helping to check us in as I was encumbered with my luggage plus the pram and the car seat. I had butterflies in my stomach as we boarded the plane with the pram, the car seat and the big baby bag. On top of the practical business of packing and storing the paraphernalia that accompanied us, I was not only nervous about flying with Zak, but also about any stares my baby would attract. I had not yet developed the tough exterior I can now display when required, and my emotions were all over the place. I came to realise that as well as any hurtful comments, we also attracted a lot of sympathy and kindness. Thankfully, on this day, the cabin crew were very helpful and the journey passed without major incident.

Years later we have become seasoned travellers and Zak takes air travel in his stride, together with the airport routines.

It was lovely to be reunited with Zak's father and the three girls. However, as I was the only one in the family to have cared for him so far, I found my protectiveness towards Zak kicking in, even amongst loved and trusted family members. The girls all wanted to play mum with him, especially when it came to feeding time. Even though Zak was now being bottle-fed, there was a knack to this and using the specialised cleft bottles and nipples had to be practised to get Zak's breathing under control, to prevent him from choking, and to ensure he had a sufficient amount of milk. He also had to be burped more as cleft babies take in more air. As much as the girls wanted to bottle feed him, I couldn't allow it. I remember India tried to pick Zak up and I rushed to stop her. 'Not like that, love,' I said, taking no notice of how her little face fell. On other occasions I had to stop myself from being over-protective and had to allow the girls, and Jake, to get involved with Zak's care.

I had missed the girls, especially India, who was now six. I noticed she'd grown a little bit and her hair was longer. I had been away from her for such a long time, and her visits to the UK had been far too brief. She was clingy and followed me around everywhere for the first few days – this hasn't changed much, even though she now lives in a different country! The girls completely adored their brother. Likewise, Zak started to bond with his three big sisters and lapped up their adoration. They were on holiday from school so we had lots of family time together.

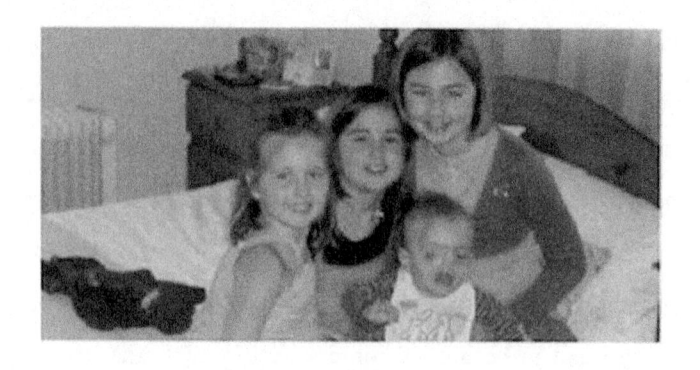

Zak and his three little mums

Cracks had already started to appear in my relationship with Jake; but our priority was Zak and the girls. There was also the worry over my mother's condition and Jake's complete disillusionment with the RAF after the way we had been abandoned by them. We both ignored the cracks, but as you can imagine, they came back to haunt us some time later.

We enjoyed the summer together as a normal family (or my version of normal) and September soon arrived. Jake's girls started a new school year, India started primary school, and Zak and I returned to the UK.

I had been told that Zak would have many check-ups and appointments during his first year of life. He remained under the eye specialist, the cleft team (including audiology, plastic surgery, speech therapy, orthodontist, and later on, a child psychologist), cardiologist and NICU, and now it was time for the first of his many surgeries.

This one was on his palate. It went extremely well and he made a quick recovery. As soon as he came round from the anaesthetic he cried for food – this was to be a regular pattern over the years as he has always loved his food, and still does. All went well and we were discharged a few days later, returning to Cyprus ten days' post-surgery.

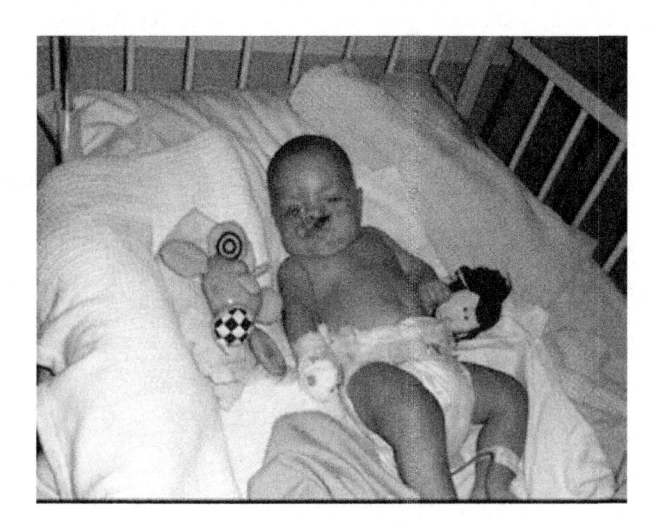

Zak, following the first operation on his palate

It was almost a full-time job to coordinate all of Zak's medical appointments but the care teams were very flexible. My brother-in-law, Glynn, took on the role of chief organiser in the UK. All of the medical letters were sent to Melanie and Glynn's home and Glynn always let me know what was going on. He scanned everything and emailed it all to me. It was like having my personal PA!

After my six months of maternity leave had finished I took nine months' unpaid leave, knowing I couldn't work and look after Zak. My sister phoned in November with bad, but not unexpected, news. My mother's condition had deteriorated and I was told that if I wanted to see her again, now was the time. Jake and I made the decision that Zak and I would travel home alone because, although India was close to my mum, I wanted her to remember her nanny at her best and it would have broken her heart if her nanny wasn't able to recognise her. I therefore told her that we were going to the UK for a number of appointments for Zak.

I saw my mum for the last time in November 2006. She was being cared for at home by Marie Curie nurses and she didn't recognise me. I said an emotional goodbye. You never think you'll lose your mum and mine was the lynchpin in our family. Not for nothing was she was known by us all as the mafia mum - if anyone upset any of her children they had better watch their back! It was only as I saw her for this last time that I realised where I got that from. The apple never falls far from the tree and that's just one of the traits I inherited from my mum.

In December 2006, Jake received an official letter from the Royal Air Force. The letter confirmed that dependency status for Zak would be granted with immediate effect, and also be backdated to his birth date. This meant that he would be treated like all other children of service personnel in Cyprus, and would therefore be entitled to the full range of medical treatment that he needed. Although Jake had submitted a formal complaint, this still came as a surprise due to their lack of compassion up to this point. The fact that it was backdated to Zak's birth was almost an insult as there was no apology or expression of regret. Due to this, our main emotion was anger because we had gone through such a traumatic time without their help when we had really needed it. We already knew they had made the wrong decision in denying Zak the treatment that other children in the same situation would be entitled to receive, and they were only doing what should have been done in the first place. So I felt little satisfaction and we did wonder whether to take legal action against the Royal Air Force.

I still held the military authorities responsible for Zak's partial blindness but did not have the emotional energy to pursue the legal avenue at that time. Fighting such a big organisation would have been emotionally draining and I wanted to put all my energy into looking after Zak and the rest of my family. This was a bitter pill to swallow.

On top of all this, my mum's condition was worsening and we all knew that she was coming to the end of her life.

My mum was legal guardian to my nephew, Kieran. She sadly passed away on his birthday, 23rd January 2007. Due to the intensive period that was my life at the time, I don't feel I was able to devote the time I needed to my mother. I've thought about this for many years since and still have feelings of guilt for not spending more time with her during her illness.

There had been some days when Zak and I were still hospital based where, although I knew I should visit mum while she was in hospital, I didn't go because Zak was either having a bad day with his saturations constantly dropping, or they had to turn up his levels on the ventilator again. So I would cancel my visit to see mum.

Looking back on this time, if I had known exactly how seriously ill mum was or how limited her time was, I would have made a different decision. Just saying that makes me feel extremely guilty - you just never know. This still haunts me some twelve years later and now I don't put things off for another day.

The times I did visit Mum in Christie's Cancer hospital were never really sad, partly because in my eyes she was having chemotherapy as a precaution/treatment, and partly because we never really knew the seriousness of her cancer: or maybe I was told and have since completely blocked it out. Perhaps it was self-preservation because at that stage of Zak's life, dealing with mum's illness would have probably sent me over the edge.

This has been the biggest regret of my life. I put Zak first before my mum. I still wonder if I was selfish in doing this or if I was just being like any other new mum with a seriously ill baby? Why didn't I try harder to split my time? Nothing I can do about it now I know, but these are questions I have asked myself over and over through the years.

My love for both my mum and my son were never in question and I'm hoping that my guilt will diminish with the passing of each year.

Mum was never an overly affectionate or demonstrative person with me and my siblings, but was completely different with her grandchildren. Saying that, we all knew that she loved us dearly. India loved her Nanny to bits. Due to my job in the travel industry I would take India back to the UK en route to a destination I needed to visit for work, and would drop her off to stay with Mum for a few days. She even had India on her first birthday because India's father and I were both away working. Many were the times India would sit with her Nanny and have a cup of tea, which always had to be in a bone china cup and saucer.

It was, however, a hard decision to make back in July, 2006. I had been given the OK to go home to my family in Cyprus for two months before Zak's first surgery in the September but at this point we all realised that Mum was extremely sick and was being looked after at home by the Macmillan nurses. My sisters both encouraged me to go home and were very supportive. I needed to be with my immediate family and hadn't really seen India properly for months. My sisters would keep me informed of any changes and update me on a regular basis. Bizarrely, when I returned to the UK that September I visited mum and for a very short period one afternoon she was lucid and sat up in bed. We had a fairly normal conversation and I secretly dared to hope that she was recovering. Now I realise that this was her final goodbye to me.

So, after Zak's surgery in September, I left again and returned to Cyprus. I received regular daily updates from both my sisters, then one day I got the call I was dreading, mum had taken a turn for the worst and maybe I should come back to say my final goodbyes. That was an extremely heartbreaking call and to this day I cannot remember if it was Shelley or Melanie that called me.

It's a very surreal feeling, being in a room with your mum knowing she is about to die. She had no awareness of me, or indeed of anyone, being there. The brain tumour was killing her but the Macmillan nurses were keeping her calm, pain-free, and sedated.

Again, my memories are very vague about the day I said goodbye. I remember the room, I remember her lying there, but I have no recollection of what I said, or how I said goodbye. Maybe I've blanked it all out. It had been a very traumatic year for me so far and looking back I'm surprised I didn't suffer more than I did. But maybe that's because I do have a very strong character and in times of crisis I can stay strong. Mum passed away peacefully at the end.

My mum loved Neil Diamond, especially the song *Sweet Caroline* which was played at her funeral. I couldn't listen to that song for years without crying and it still brings a tear to my eye when I hear it now. My sisters feel exactly the same.

*****

Zak's next operation was in February 2007, prior to his first birthday which he spent in hospital. This one was to repair part of his palate.

Because Zak's cleft was extremely rare, the medical team wanted to feature him in their Medical Journal and this became the first of many media appearances for my son. I signed a form agreeing they could take photographs during and post surgery and this is what happened, with Zak knowing little about what was going on.

Like most things in his life, when he was old enough to understand, he took to media attention like a duck to water.

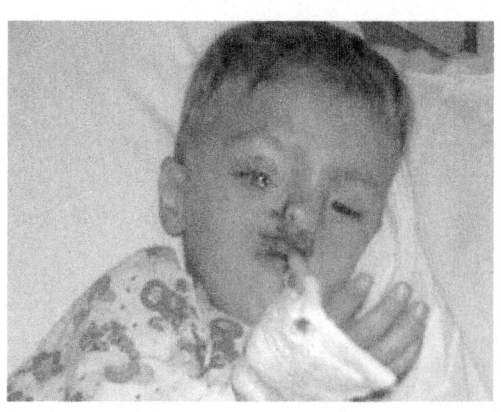

Following another operation to repair Zak's palate

Zak was formally discharged from the NICU and cardiology shortly after his first birthday and this turning point meant we had to prepare for the further operations he'd require before his second.

His third surgery was to repair the side of his nostril and top lip.

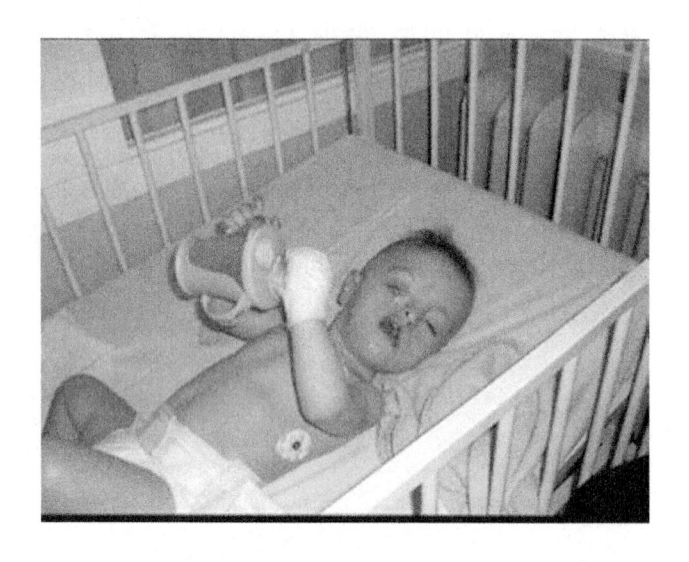

Post operation – Zak's more than ready for some food!

The fourth involved inserting a tissue expander. This is a small flat balloon which went under the skin behind Zak's ear. We needed to stay in the UK for two months while this was carried out as we had to return to the hospital on a weekly basis, for six weeks, so that a saline solution could be inserted into the balloon in order for it to inflate and for his skin to grow around it. This would give the surgeons excess skin to work with to be able to reconstruct a new lower eyelid.

Zak attracted many strange looks during this time due to the balloon growing on the side of his face. It wasn't easy by any means. Zak was becoming a clumsy toddler and I had to control his movements to ensure the balloon was not damaged while he was running around. One day the balloon didn't look right to me and felt hot to the touch. With a mother's instincts, I knew he'd contracted an infection, and I was proven right when I took Zak to be checked and he was taken straight into A&E and put onto powerful antibiotics. I was told that if they didn't work, they would have to remove the balloon and start all over again with a new balloon, at a later date. We all kept our fingers crossed and, thankfully, the situation improved the next day, the antibiotics having done their job.

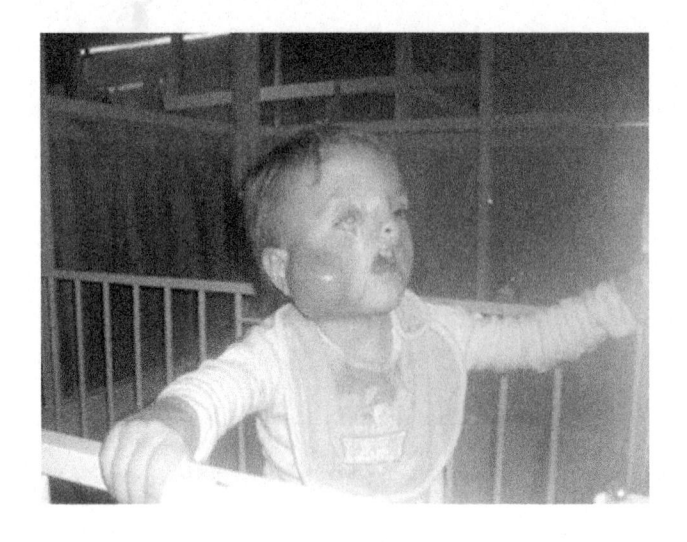

Zak with his tissue expander

The operation went ahead six weeks after the balloon had been inserted. Both the balloon and the excess skin were removed and the surgeons started their work to construct the right side of Zak's face. This was a very complex surgery involving construction of his cheek, his lower eyelid and lip. Three surgeons worked on my son during this surgery. I stayed overnight on the cleft lip and palate ward where we had a bedsit type setup. There were also other facilities for the parents, such as a communal kitchen, bathroom and sitting room with TV. They tended to operate on babies as early in the day as possible and my worry was always that Zak was unable to eat for a while before his operations. A major task was trying to keep his mind off food prior to the operations which I did by playing with him or chattering about everything. Even so, he was always upset not to be able to have his first bottle in the morning.

After putting his gown on, signing the consent form and carrying Zak, I accompanied the nurses to the anaesthetic room. 'Are you okay, Mum?' one of the nurses asked as I looked around the room at the anaesthetist, three nurses, and plastic surgeon.

'I'm fine,' I replied crying as I did so.

'Are all the details correct?' the anaesthetist asked while looking at Zak's notes. I said they were and he explained what would happen next. I watched as they put a mask on Zak to send him to sleep. One of the nurses touched my arm and gave a gentle smile.

'Come on,' she said, and I followed them back to the ward and went to my bedsit where I spent my time alternately pacing up and down or sitting and staring at the walls. Fed up with driving myself nuts, I went for a shower to try and take my mind off the operation. It didn't work but at least I was clean! I knew the operation was going to be at least six hours so I phoned Jake, then Melanie, and eventually a nurse came to take me to the recovery room.

'All has gone well but we will need to monitor him in ICU,' she said. I had already been informed that this would happen, so I grabbed his comfort blankets and we made our way there.

Following the operation, Zak was monitored in intensive care overnight. We knew all was well when he woke up and, true to form, immediately asked for food. I was able to give him a bottle and then he went to sleep.

After spending the rest of the day and some of the night with Zak, a nurse said, 'Go back to your room and have a sleep.' Knowing Zak was out of danger, I made my way back to our bedsit on the ward. By now it was the dead of night. The route back to the bedsit was along a long and dark corridor. I had been told this area was haunted and as I started to walk, I heard creaks and groans from the building that I wasn't accustomed to. My imagination went into overdrive and I sprinted as if being chased by the devil's hounds. I felt a little silly when I jumped onto my bed out of breath a few minutes later!

Zak recovered very quickly and was discharged shortly after, the surgery having been a complete success. Due to the fact that Zak now had a partial lower eyelid, the scar tissue surrounding it was able to decrease. However, even though the operation was a success, Zak is, even now, unable to fully close his eye. Whilst he is able to distinguish between light and dark, he will never have proper vision and will remain blind in his right eye.

When Zak was eighteen months old, Jake's daughters went to live with their mother in the UK. This coincided with Lucy, the oldest, starting senior school. I was sad to see them go but didn't have a choice in the matter. The four children had always got along very well and missed each other when Lucy and Hannah left.

For the first two years of Zak's life we travelled back and forth to the UK to attend his many appointments and surgeries. He'd had four surgeries by the time he was two years old.

I'm not a particularly religious person but Zak had been baptized when I was unconscious after my emergency C-section and I felt that I'd missed out on an important event in his life. He had already come a long way in his short life and we, as a family, wanted to celebrate this. I was determined to have a massive celebration of Zak's life.

We went to see the Chaplain at St Barnabas Church in Limassol. We explained our situation and he smiled sympathetically.

'Zak has already been officially baptized,' he said, 'but all is not lost.'

We were told that the only other option would be for a naming ceremony which was a similar ceremony.

We set the date and I planned it with military precision... ohh how coincidental!

All overseas visitors and guests started to arrive a couple of days prior to the ceremony so we had a full very busy house. My sister Melanie and her family, Jake's mum Dorothy, my best friend, Liz, and Zak's sisters, Lucy &

Hannah. In total, we invited 25 guests.

On the morning of the ceremony it was an extremely busy house with all five girls (India, Lucy, Hannah, Hope and Robyn) to get ready. You can imagine how busy the two bathrooms were. Robyn and Lucy took charge and did all the girls' hair and minimal makeup. Zak was aware there was a party but no idea what for, he just went along with the flow and became extremely excited. India, Hannah and Hope all had matching outfits - floral pink skirts with white vests – and they looked absolutely adorable.

Zak was very dapper in his linen blue shorts and matching waistcoat, with crisp white linen shirt (which didn't stay crisp for very long).

I remember it was a beautiful sunny day with temperatures of about twenty-five degrees.

The ceremony was in the British Church and such was the atmosphere and surroundings, we felt as if we could have been in a British country village on a beautiful summer's day. Zak was such a good boy for the most part, though he had to be restrained at one point from running up and down the aisle. The day was all about him, and although he was too young to fully understand, he definitely picked up on positive vibes and the joyous mood of the day.

My emotions were mixed. I felt so blessed that my son had come through what he had and was growing into a lovely young lad and it was a pleasure to share such a special day with loved family and friends. But there was also a tinge of sadness that I had missed Zak's baptism.

The after party was at the Hotel Miramare in Limassol. The setting was picturesque, beside the pool/fish ponds adjacent to the beach, and we were served a lovely sit down meal by wonderfully attentive waiters.

Zak changed his outfit post ceremony into his Manchester United kit.... courtesy of Uncle Glynn and Auntie Melanie. This caused some friendly banter due to the fact that Jake is a Sunderland supporter.

It was a fabulous day from start to finish. A true celebration of Zak's life and name.

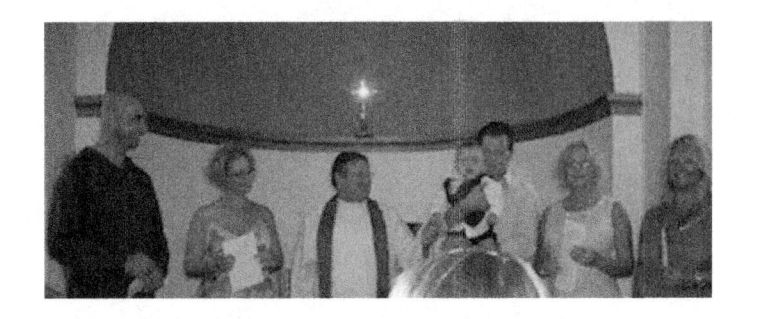

The Naming Ceremony – happy days!

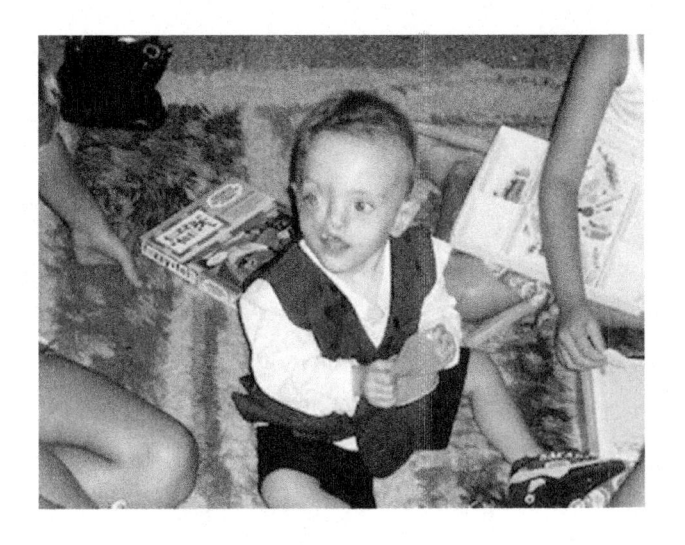

How cute does he look?

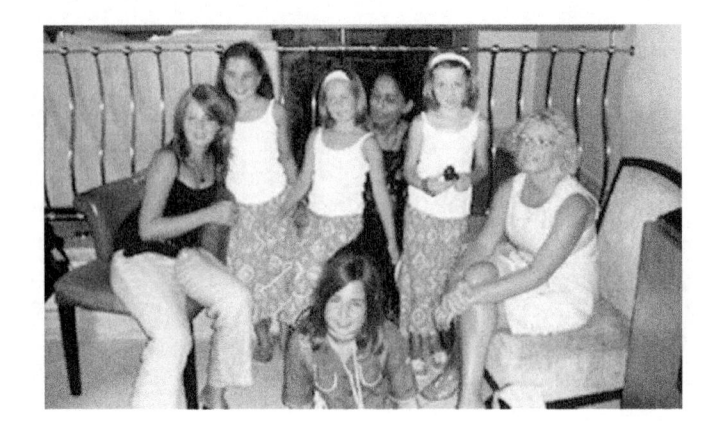

The ladies, all ready to go

(I remember Zak's Godmother, Liz, telling me some time later, 'Zak is a strong, determined and engaging young man, who I've had the pleasure of knowing all of his life. It's an honour to be Zak's godmother, and to see him continue to grow in every way each year! I wish Zak all the luck in the world.')

By now, my nine-month's unpaid leave had turned into two years - the first two of Zak's life. The years had flown by and it was time for me to return to work. My company went through a reshuffle while I was pregnant and I had been promoted to regional manager. Returning to work at this elevated level was the worst decision I ever made, but we're all great with hindsight, aren't we? There was lots of travel involved which meant I had to spend time away from my family – something I hadn't thought through prior to accepting the raise in status. I didn't enjoy the new job and was desperate to be at home. I'd changed from being a career-focussed individual to a mother who worried about time spent away from her kids.

My company merged with another shortly after and I was able to change my lifestyle by accepting voluntary redundancy in September 2008. This was absolutely the right decision for me and it came at exactly the right time. I took two years out where I tried various projects, one of which was taking a course to learn how to work with children with ADHD. I learnt a lot but decided this wasn't the career for me. I also looked into becoming a salesperson, selling air-cooling mist systems. Again, this wasn't for me and came to nothing.

A further complication for Zak during the first two years of his life was his lungs and difficulty with breathing. Due to his prematurity and the fact that he was on a ventilator to help him breathe for the first three months, he developed chronic lung disease. Lungs can regenerate over time but in someone so small it takes longer. The result of this was that Zak was admitted to hospital seven times during this period, suffering from either bronchitis or bronchial pneumonia. He also had to use a nebulizer (a device used to administer medication in the form of a mist inhaled into the lungs. Nebulizers are commonly used for the treatment of asthma, cystic fibrosis, COPD and other respiratory diseases or disorders) or inhaler on a regular basis.

When he was two, Zak started nursery. This gave the family a sense of normality – at least, as far as the children were concerned. He soon made lots of new friends and has continued to do so, ever since. Two of his earliest, Pavlo and Emily, he is friends with to this day, some eleven years later.

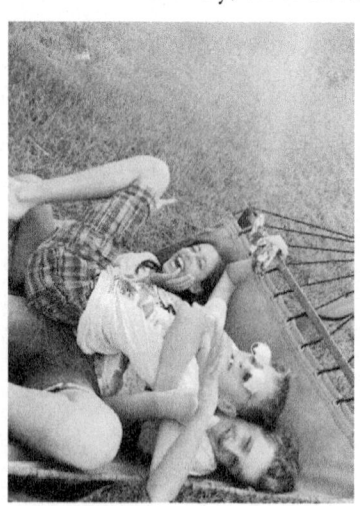

Zak and his forever friends, Pavlo and Emily

I'm not sure if it was then or a little earlier that we all realised Zak was going to be a chatterbox, and also a very determined little boy. He was constantly on the naughty step from this age forward for about two years. When Zak refused to do something, such as finishing his dinner, moving his clothes or food bowls, or generally not listening to what I said, I started to use the phrase, 'I'm disappointed with you, Zak, go and sit on the naughty step.' This became such a regular occurrence that Zak got into the habit of taking himself off to the naughty step without having to be told to do so!

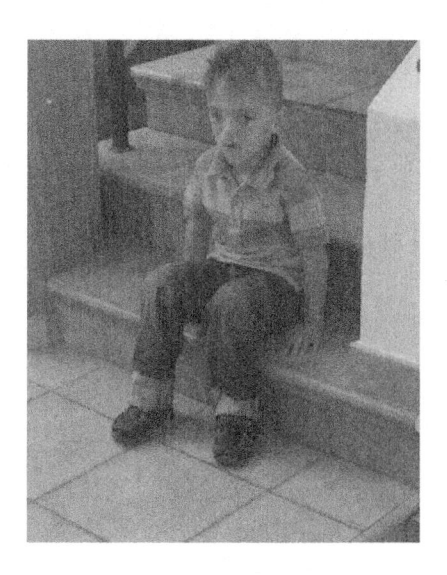

On the naughty step – again!

'I'm going to sit on the step,' he'd say.

I would respond by saying, 'Go and think about what you've done.' It hardly seemed like a punishment though as Zak would sit there singing to himself, in his own little world. And when he was a little older, I discovered he could see the television from the naughty step…

I also used the counting method. 'I'm going to count to three, Zak, then you'll be in trouble.' I have reached two and a half but never three, and I have never had to shout at Zak who gets upset when I use the phrase 'I'm disappointed with you.'

From a very young age his outgoing personality has shone through. He loves to dress up and will talk to anyone about anything, no matter their age, background or experience.

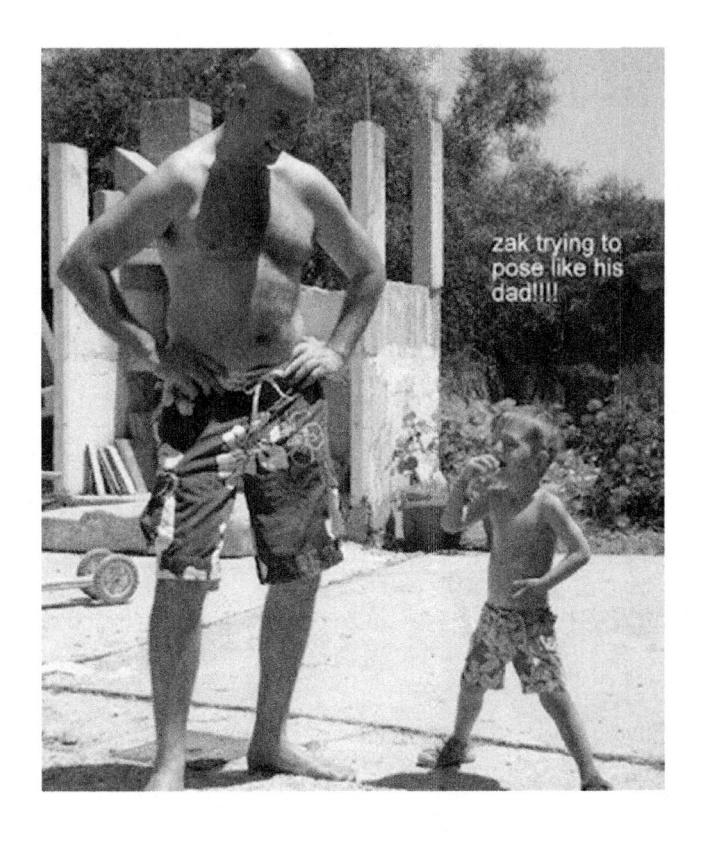

Zak, trying to pose like his dad!

Down to Business

Zak was approaching four years old when I set up a medical tourism business along with two other friends. Medical tourism was the new craze as people realised that it wasn't just celebrities who wanted to look the best that they could, and the decrease in prices meant it was now affordable to many. All three of us had worked in the travel industry for many years, so we saw the opportunity and went for it. Before joining the travel industry, I was a dental nurse and I loved that job but struggled to get on with one of the staff, which led me to a change of career. I have been asked many times since whether I made this career choice because of Zak's condition and the answer is no, but I do believe in helping people to be the best version of themselves where I can. In addition, having spent so many months in hospitals with Zak, I had the knowledge and experience of how some processes work. Knowledge I have gained since starting the business has also allowed me to help Zak with pain relief and post-surgery care. I should point out here that I am not medically trained, what I have learned has come purely from my experience of looking after my child; as any mother with a child in hospital knows, you become the main carer (effectively an untrained proxy nurse).

Zak's surgeries were carried out by the Consultant Plastic Surgeons, Mr Peter Davenport and Miss Victoria Beale, and the Opthalmic Plastic Surgeons, Mr Brian Leatherbarrow and Ms Anne Cook. Every operation has been carried out at Booth Hall Hospital (which has now been amalgamated to become Manchester Children's Hospital) and we have been made to feel part of the family there. As well as giving Zak first-class treatment and after care, my family and I have been treated with warmth, compassion and kindness. We have to travel between Cyprus and the UK for all hospital visits/operations/follow-up checks and any other appointments, and everything has been excellent.

Zak was aged four and five when he had operations six and seven, and these were minor compared to those he'd already been through. These operations changed the appearance of his upper lip; he was undergoing speech therapy at this stage. He remained his happy go lucky self, and still loved dressing up in whatever took his fancy at the time.

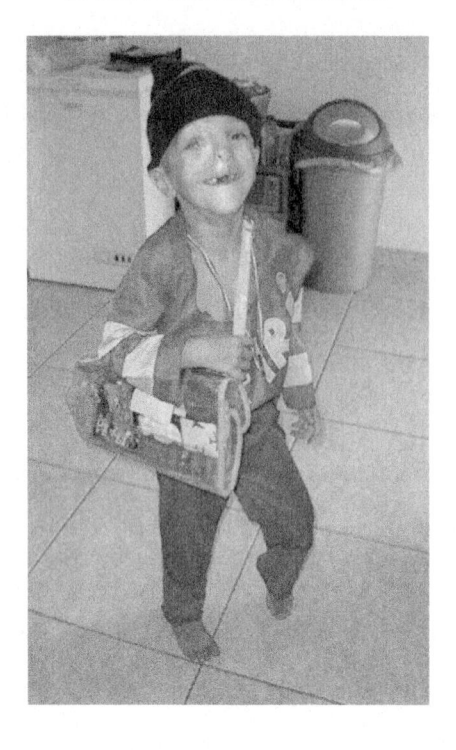

Zak's fancy dress – just because he can!

Following twenty-four years of service, Jake left the Royal Air Force and came back to civvy street. He became a contractor for the Ministry of Defence, in Episkopi, Cyprus. The stress, upset, and anger over the way they had treated us took its toll and we looked again into the possibility of taking legal action against the Air Force. Jake spent many hours putting together a case file and he spoke to a UK lawyer who was confident that we had a strong case. However, this was all still very emotionally draining for us both and was too much to deal with when trying to look after the children, so we decided to put it on hold.

The routine of family life continued with India starting senior school in 2011 and Zak, primary. Lucy and Hannah visited us that summer and there was a big family outing to take Zak, aged six, to school. Zak was mega excited. He didn't want any of us to go into the playground but we followed him anyway, all of us taking photos like the proud parents and sisters we were.

I was worried that Zak would be bullied due to his looks. India was due to start senior school which was at the same location where she had attended primary - this was a big international school and I didn't particularly want Zak to go somewhere so big. After India and I chatted about it, she asked whether she could attend a smaller senior school with Zak in the primary where she could keep an eye on him. This was an ideal solution and it made me feel better, knowing his big sister would be there should anyone decide to pick on him. So India switched schools and Zak went to his classroom and India to hers. When I went to pick him up at the end of his school day, he was fine - but he told me later that a Russian girl had approached him in the playground and called him a monster. My insides immediately knotted and it was all I could do to stop myself screaming at the cruelty of some people. I managed to hide my feelings from Zak and asked how he had responded. Zak didn't seem particularly bothered and I laughed when he told me he had pulled a face at the girl and she ran away screaming. This incident made me decide to speak to the teachers to discuss how the school intended to deal with this kind of behaviour and how to explain Zak's facial differences. I took some 'Lippy the Lion' books, which tell a story about a baby lion with a cleft lip, and the teachers used these to show the children why Zak was different. I know that children (and adults) are curious about people who look different, and while it's human nature, it is not necessary to be cruel. The point of taking the books in and speaking to the teachers was to try to educate them that although Zak looks unique, it does not give anyone the right to be cruel or unkind. We're all different in one way or another, and those who are unique shouldn't be punished or ridiculed because of the way they look.

dailymail.co.uk ✕

☰ **Mail**Online Health

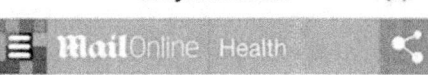

He's been called a 'monster' and stared at by strangers - but little boy with severe cleft lip has just one response - he SMILES back

By Lizzie Parry for MailOnline
17:26 10 Sep 2015, updated 08:26 11 Sep 2015

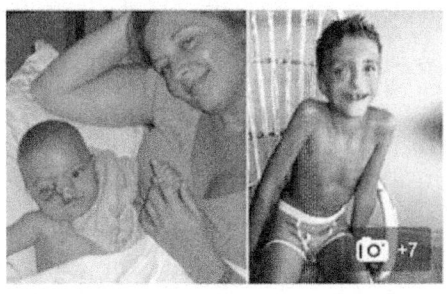

One of the many articles featuring Zak

Because he is blind in one eye, Zak struggled with school right from the start. He's right handed, which means that because he can't see from his right eye it is hard for him to hold a pencil or to co-ordinate his actions whilst holding it. It has taken a lot of work and patience from both Zak and his teachers in order for him to be able to do this properly.

Zak showed an interest in history from a young age and is fascinated by many people from the past. Florence

Nightingale was his first love, hearing her story not long after he started primary school. When my friend, Julie, visited she was fascinated by Zak carrying around a picture. 'What's that?' she asked.

'You mean who,' Zak replied, showing Julie the picture of Florence Nightingale. He then regaled her with tales of Florence's life as if she had been a personal friend, until satisfied that Julie was now properly educated on everything to do with Florence.

I remember Julie telling me, "This wonderfully witty, intelligent, fun-loving boy is very special."

(During a later visit by Julie, Zak had moved on from Florence Nightingale and was now obsessed by ants. As she arrived he asked her to sit down and watch various You Tube videos about ants and their nests. The following morning he woke her at 6 am. Both in pyjamas, they went hunting for an ant's nest. Julie wasn't allowed to return home until she could identify the Queen Ant!)

Our lives were a whirlwind as Zak and I had to travel to the UK frequently for his various appointments.

Unfortunately, he had begun to suffer from a number of eye infections in his left eye and required a CT scan which showed that he didn't have a tear duct system in his left eye, but he did in his right – his blind eye. So the next operation was for Zak to be given an artificial tear duct system, and this one took place in the Ocular Plastic department at Manchester Eye Hospital. Before the operation took place, the consultant told me that Zak would need to keep a patch over his eye for a few days following the operation. I was most uncomfortable with this news as it would effectively make him completely blind, albeit temporarily. My heart went out to my little man as I knew this would throw him into a panic and make him unhappy. I told the consultant but he insisted that the patch would have to remain in place. However, Zak was completely distraught when he came round from the anaesthetic and kept pulling at the patch. The medical staff were worried that this would adversely affect his new tear duct system so they agreed that the patch could be removed on condition that I kept vigil at Zak's bedside to ensure that he didn't touch his eye. This was a good compromise and Zak immediately calmed down and became his usual post-op self; he asked for some food.

Thankfully, Zak healed very well from this operation and has had no further eye infections.

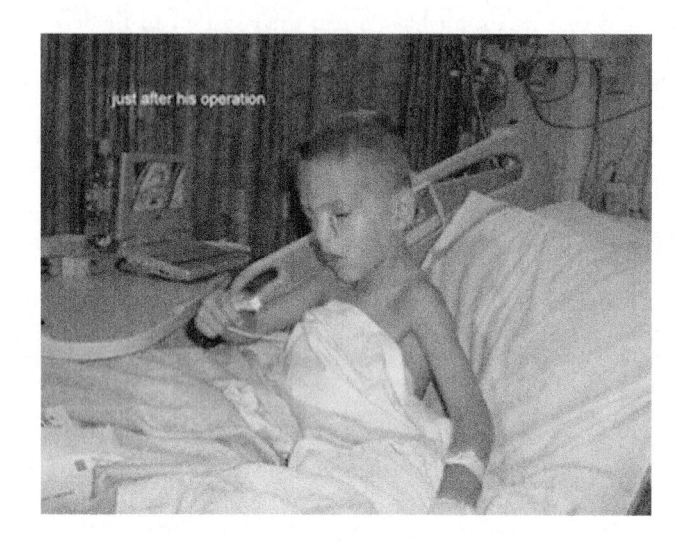

Zak after receiving an artificial tear duct system

Single Mum

At the beginning of 2012, Jake decided to accept an offer of work as a contractor in Afghanistan. Following that, he took a job at the London Olympics. We were living separate lives and the cracks that had started to appear earlier in our relationship were now massive fissures. He returned to Cyprus about a month after the Olympic Games finished, and we made the decision to split.

So began my time as a second-time single mum. Jake returned to the UK and India, Zak and I became a relaxed and happy family unit.

During Jake's visit before Christmas 2013 we decided to have a family day in Troodos. We were all in for a surprise when we saw a VIP surrounded by his entourage of close protection policemen and other staff.

'Look, there's the President of Cyprus,' I whispered, and pointed to the group who were within hearing distance.

'I want to meet him,' Zak said, and rushed off before we had a chance to stop him.

Jake and I hurried to follow as we watched one of the President's close protection team attempt to block Zak's access to the president. The President said something to the policeman and then encouraged Zak to approach. I quickly took out my phone and took a snap. President Nicos Anastasiades was a true gentleman and made a wonderful day even better!

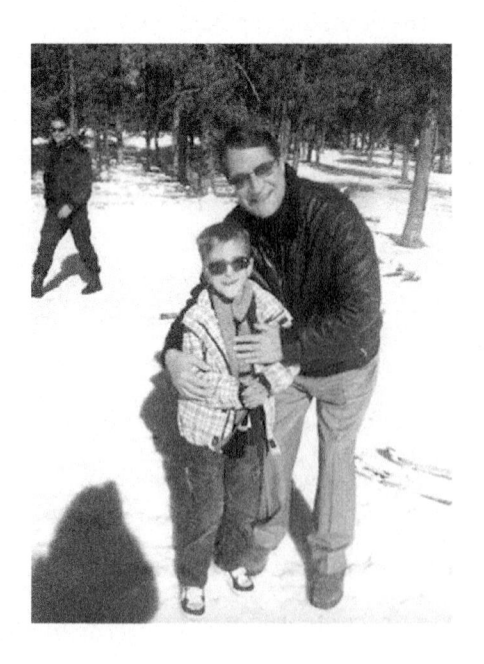

Hello Mr President!

Before Zak's next surgery, we had a trip down memory lane and revisited the NICU Unit. The photos are with some of the NICU Team and Zak's Neo Natal Consultant.

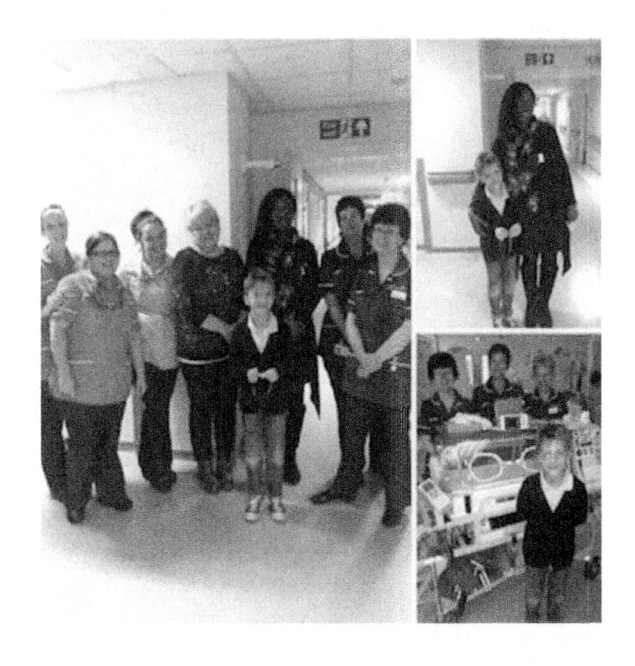

With the wonderful life-saving team!

Zak's next surgery was to widen his palate and to fit a permanent brace. This treatment was needed to enable him to have a bone graft later on, as bone was missing due to the cleft. Without this, his adult teeth would not be able to erupt.

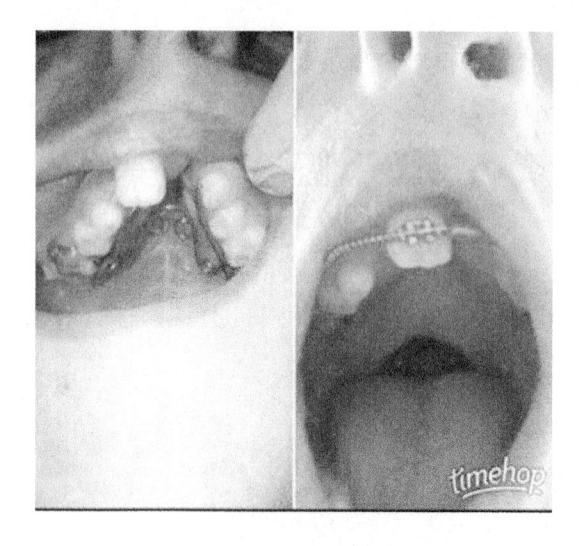

Then and now

Zak's bone graft surgery (Alveolar Bone Graft (ABG)) was completed towards the end of 2015 when he was nine years old. This was another major operation where the surgeon had to remove bone from Zak's hip and implant it into his gum above his top lip. His second teeth were ready to come through but there was nothing for them to fix onto.

I was told to expect a long recovery period and that Zak would struggle to walk because of what was done to his hip. During the procedure, bone marrow is taken from the hip and grafted into the gap left by the cleft. It is usually approximately a five-centimetre long cut over the hip bone with the surgeon going into the bone and scooping out the inner marrow, hence the pain and long recovery period. The bone marrow is then packed into the pocket within the gum and stitched up. It can take up to two years for the newly placed bone marrow to develop.

I was told that children who undergo this operation generally have massively swollen faces afterwards. However, even though his face was swollen, thirty minutes after he had woken up, Zak said he was starving and demanded food. The medical staff were very impressed with his recovery and allowed him to walk (very slowly) to the hospital canteen where one of the ladies made him his favourite tuna sandwiches. He wolfed them down like he hadn't eaten for a month!

We spent two weeks in the UK leading both up to and following this operation. This was to be the last surgery for a while until we were informed whether the bone graft was considered to be successful or not. Two years later, we were told that it had worked (though it was four years before the first tooth came through) and were informed that the next stage of Zak's treatment would be for his eye reconstruction.

To date, a team from the Eye Hospital have met with specialists from around the UK to discuss the best way forward. Zak's bottom eyelid still needs further treatment because he is unable to close his eye. In addition, the position of Zak's nose needs to be corrected and specialists are currently working on the best way to do this. Zak is due a review soon when they will give us the plan for his future surgeries.

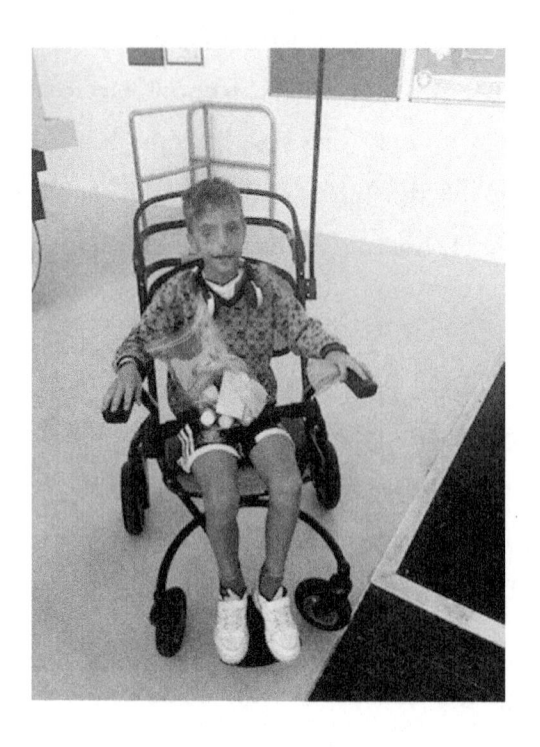

Zak after his bone graft surgery

Zak was going through his Zombie Apocalypse fascination round about the time of his bone graft surgery. When he first started talking about what would happen should there be a Zombie Apocalypse it was quite amusing, but it ended up driving us all nuts!

Some of the older visitors to Lenia's, the local village tavern, were bemused by Zak's serious questions about what they intended to do when (*yes, when, and not if*) it happened, and how they planned to get away from the Zombies. However, they did enjoy his anecdotes and facts about other historical characters and information about the lives and habits of many animals.

Lenia's is less than a five minute walk from our home, and we often meet friends there for a drink or some delicious food. You can guarantee that on a Friday night Molly (a very senior lady) will be there, sometimes Andy (not quite as senior) and perhaps Lili and Derek, Deb and Allan, and Dean and Sarah.

I remember Zak running ahead of India on a balmy Friday evening when I'd decided to treat the kids to dinner at

Lenia's. As India and I approached, we watched him high five my eclectic group of friends and by the time we arrived, the discussion about the forthcoming Zombie Apocalypse was well under way.

'So, Molly, you need to store as many tins as you can because the last thing you want is to run out of food.'

'But I don't eat that much, Zak.' Molly nodded to her half eaten meal she always referred to as *chips and egg*, her regular Friday evening meal.

'But what if you're hungry and you haven't got any food? You can't take egg and chips with you,' Zak said, addressing the whole table before rolling his eyes as if they didn't understand the simplest of instructions.

'So where are you going to hide, Zak, and where do you suggest we hide?' asked Derek, practical as ever.

'Good question, Derek,' said Zak. 'I'm glad someone is taking this seriously.' With that he took a piece of paper out of his pocket and laid it flat on the table next to Derek. Zak had drawn a rough sketch of the waste ground next to our home where he intended to build the bunker. There was a sleeping area, a storeroom and a small relaxation area.

'And where will we go to wash and...'

Zak interrupted Lili. 'When the Zombie Apocalypse happens, I don't think you'll be worried about washing,' he replied. 'Mum, can I have some money to play pool?'

I happily handed over a euro. Zak picked up his bunker plan and folded it back in his pocket, then ran off to find someone to play pool with and no doubt, to discuss the forthcoming apocalypse with them.

'That boy's going to go places,' said Molly, laughing. 'You mark my words.'

Shortly after this, Derek presented Zak with a book entitled: *How to Survive the Zombie Apocalypse*. To say my son was delighted with this gift was a major understatement.

On another occasion, Deb and her husband Allan looked after Zak for a day while I took India on an outing. They told me later that he *interviewed* them about their entire lives together and they felt as if they were part of a TV show at one stage. They took him for tea at the tavern and as they left the house Zak asked, 'How long have you been together?'

'Forever, Zak,' Deb answered.

'No, really?'

'She's right. Or it seems like forever, anyway.'

'That's unkind, Allan, and not very nice,' Zak replied although he did laugh. 'So where did you meet and what made you get together?'

'We met in Scotland and we liked each other straight away.'

'What did you first like about each other?'

'Good grief, Zak!' said Deb.

'Okay, okay. Well how long have you been in Cyprus and what made you want to live here? When do you think the Zombie Apocalypse will happen? There won't be many survivors. We've already started storing tins and stuff to take to the bunker.'

They enjoyed Zak's company so much that they encouraged me to leave him with them again! I'm very proud that Zak is so entertaining and such an extrovert.

Things could have been very different, especially here in Cyprus where disabled or different children are often hidden away in the rural villages. Those that aren't hidden have to endure stares, and in some instances, blatant comments about their differences. This happened to us in Zak's favourite restaurant, Pizza Express.

We used to go to Pizza Express with Pavlos and Emily and their parents some Sundays when the restaurant had a clown to entertain the children. It was always packed and our favourite place to sit was upstairs.

As we walked in, instead of the buzz and bustle of a busy restaurant, I felt a silence. A few adults and children stared but this seemed to have a domino effect and soon after, it felt like everyone who could see us, was staring at us. A few children even ran away from the clown, back to where their parents were sitting. At this point in our lives I was still extremely sensitive and outraged by this reaction, even though Zak, Pavlos, and Emily were completely oblivious to what was going on. We still ate there and the kids had fun but it put a massive dampener on my day and my fury didn't subside. I wrote to the Cyprus Sunday Mail telling them what had happened and emphasising the fact that people with differences are (for the most part) hidden away in Cyprus. Because of this, some Cypriots are cruel and insensitive. The paper published my letter the following week. Some time later, 'Pick Me Up!' magazine contacted me and wrote the following article:

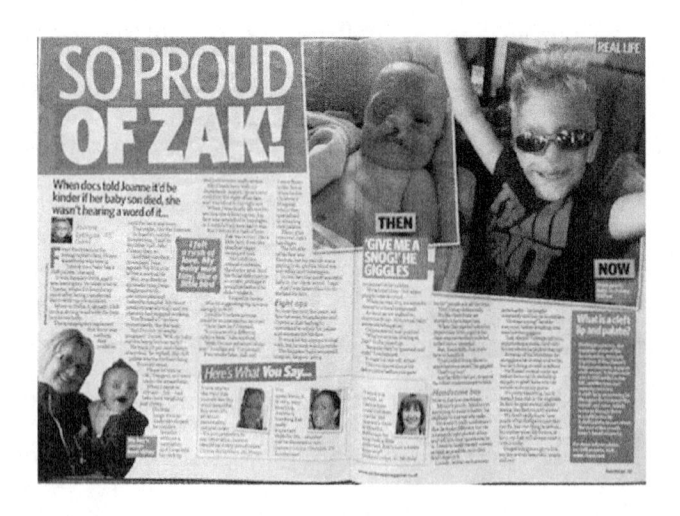

My little media star!

As a result of this, a number of other publications contacted me. Zak has since appeared in numerous magazines/newspapers and quite enjoys the attention.

He's also keen for people to know that although his cleft makes him unique, he's just a boy who loves life and loves spending time with his friends and family – the same as other boys.

A woman named Andrea contacted me from Slovakia in 2016, telling me that Zak was an inspiration to her and her family. She explained that her son was due to be born in October and had already been diagnosed with the same rare cleft as Zak. She asked me many questions and looked at all Zak's photographs and I told her about the surgeries. In her own words, she said, '*It's been a great inspiration for me and has made me and my husband very optimistic about the future for when our baby is born.*' She went on to say that they intended to name their baby boy Zak, after my little boy wonder. Little Zak was born on 15 September 2016.

Did I mention that Zak loves animals? We currently have two dogs and two and a half cats (the half is because one decides to spend some of the time with us and some with a Russian family who live a few streets away!). Lola, our Pug, and Zak have been best friends since we bought her from the pet shop in 2011. We only went there for fish food and came home £CY700 lighter in the purse, with a puppy! The arrival of Obie, our rescue dog, hasn't changed Zak and Lola's friendship, but has added to it. Obie's an escape artist and Zak is often called on to chase him around the village and bring him home. No matter how much we try to 'Obie proof' the garden, he always seems to find a space to wriggle through.

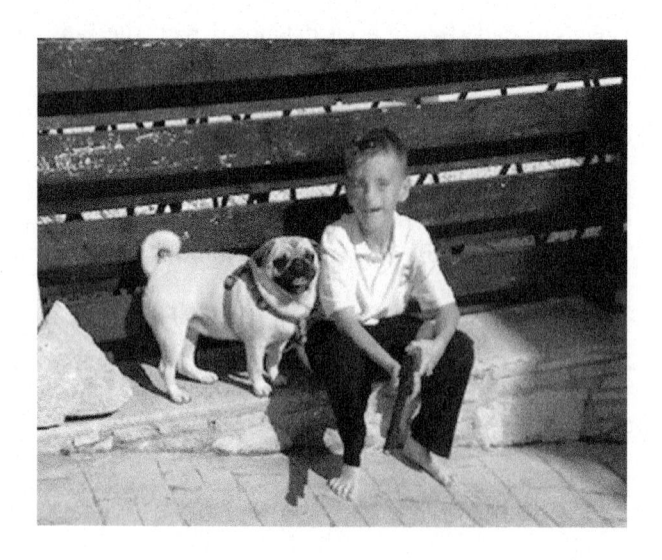

With best friend, Lola

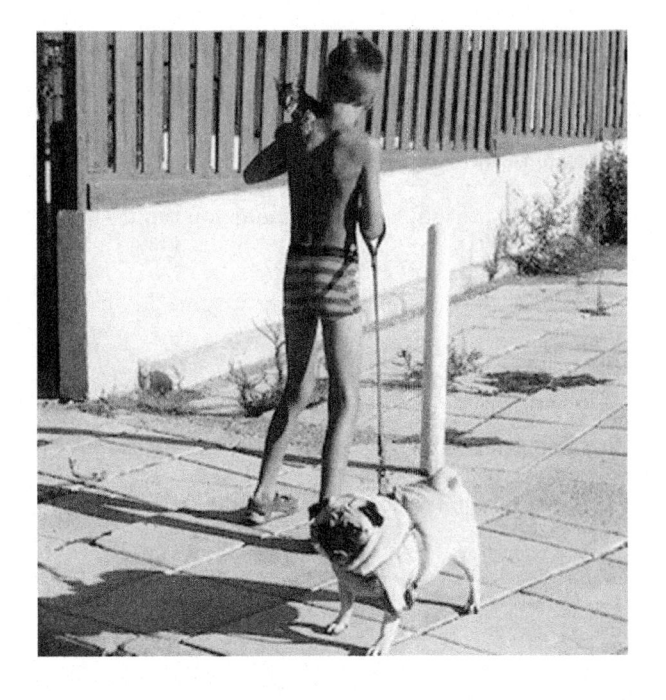

Dressing down to take the pets for a walk

Zak started senior school in September 2017 and has extra help with maths. As Zak hates the subject, I don't believe this is anything to do with his condition, any more than any other children who hate maths. India is something of a maths legend, so she tutors him and he has made vast improvements. India wrote an algebra test for Zak, following a tutoring session on this subject. 'Ready for this, Zak?' she asked, putting the papers down in front of him.

Zak's response was to stare at his sister then at the papers, the latter with an expression of confusion on his face. I can recall India sighing before saying, 'Just try your best, Zak. We've been through all of this and you can do it.'

He stared at the papers again and his sister then became irritated. 'Just get on with it!'

I intervened at this point and Zak ended up crying with frustration before leaving the room in a huff.

Despite India's best efforts, this was the usual scenario.

My friend Liz, is also a maths guru and has helped Zak immensely. However, he dreads it when Liz is due to visit purely because of the extra maths classes! On the flip side of the coin, Zak is extremely knowledgeable about, indeed obsessed with, social history and some of the people who are long since dead. He surprised me by following the news of the death of Stan Lee, the famous illustrator of Marvel Books. Zak's current passion is comic illustrations and when Mr Lee's death was announced, my son reeled off his life and career achievements as if he had known him personally.

So, all in all, our lives have completely changed. We have a son who both Jake and I are immensely proud of. We have had to become strong when people stare at Zak in public. When he was younger, I was very defensive and used to question people for staring; now I retaliate less, understanding that it is human nature and people stare because Zak looks different. Having been told he is beautiful since very young, Zak is a happy and confident child. Although his speech was delayed due to the cleft and surgeries, this has never stopped him from trying to talk. He was a toddler when he first said '…'ummy', and it brought tears to my eyes because, due to the structure of his mouth, it was difficult for Zak to make certain sounds and one was the 'em' sound. It's not been a problem since.

Zak's sisters and cousins love him to bits and are very protective of him. Once they get past his unusual looks, anyone who meets Zak comes to love his happy, infectious nature.

Zak started to become aware of the fact that he looks different when he was about five years old. One day he asked, 'Mummy, why does my eye look different?'

'That's just the way you are, Zak,' I replied. 'But the doctors are going to make your eye better.'

From then on, if anyone asked Zak any questions about his differences, his standard response was that the doctors were going to make him better. Strangely, he has never asked about his lip, or the rest of his face. I have always taught my son that being unique is a good thing and to embrace who you are. The Dr Seuss quote at the beginning of this book has been our motto, *"Why fit in when you were born to stand out?"* and for Zak these differences have never been a major issue.

Zak loves drawing and when a psychologist saw the picture of an avatar that he created (with the help of a computer programme), she commented that he must be confident for his avatar to be what most would consider imperfect. I explained that Zak has never shied away from looking in the mirror and is confident about the way he looks. He's happy to take selfies from his blind side and if we're on holiday, will always get up on stage if a performer asks for a volunteer.

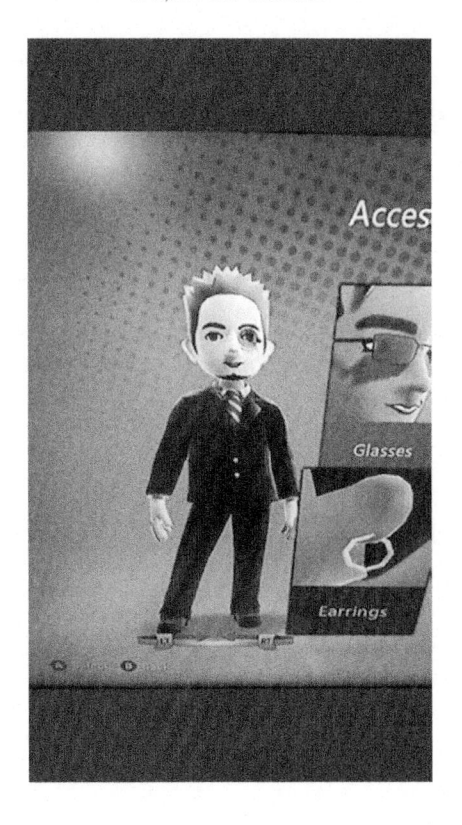

Zak's avatar

Zak has an instant empathy with anyone who looks different, and he's never afraid to speak up for the underdog if he sees somebody being picked on, or bullied. I'm pretty chuffed that my son has such an outgoing, extrovert, personality, despite, or maybe because of, everything he's been through.

As I write (2019), Zak's first tooth has appeared through his bone graft. The surgery was some four years ago. This graft has now been deemed a success and his next operations will be to complete the reconstruction of his bottom eyelid. As always, Zak takes all of his operations in his stride, and hopefully this won't change now that he's growing up.

The Big Picture

Although this is Zak's story, his life, my own, and India's are all intertwined, together with those of our families and close friends. I've included some of their thoughts and anecdotes in this chapter.

India is now grown up and has recently started university in Liverpool. She and Zak miss each other but FaceTime to tease one another and for India to nag her little brother.

When I asked India for her comments she said, 'He's a pain in the backside!' After laughing about this, she added, 'When I was younger it used to upset me when people stared and I felt very protective and often fought his corner. Although he's sometimes an annoying little brother I love him and miss him now that I've moved away from home.'

In the early years we spent more time with Melanie, Glynn, Robyn and Hope, than we did at home in Cyprus. We all have many memories of both the good and also the difficult times. Talking to Melanie about this the other day she said, 'Looking back, we all just got on with it, and having you and Zak living with us was good because we all got on so well. Robyn and Hope never moaned once about having to give up their bedrooms and they always made me proud how very protective they were when people would stare at him because he looked different. It's been a pleasure being able to help you both when it must have been so difficult with Zak in hospital in Manchester, and India in school in Cyprus. I'm just so glad we could help. I think we all have a special kind of love for Zak because we have been such a big part of his early years. He is a total credit to you now that he is a very caring young boy with a great personality which will help him with any obstacles he has to face in the future.'

Glynn added, 'Having family stay with us is always a pleasure and we all always look forward to you coming to stay with us. Watching Zak grow and become the cool and thoughtful person he is today has been a joy.

'He has, through the years, been a character with a strong determination. I remember him borrowing an Apple charger and then when he was leaving he was adamant it was his.... little loveable lad and the house was always lively when he was here with his Nerf gun bullets flying everywhere or drones hitting the lights. But Mel was always the laid back sister (said tongue in cheek!) and took it in her stride. He is a credit to Jo and such a caring young man. When Mel was over in Cyprus for an operation, Zak looked after her!'

Robyn said, 'I have loved having you all here and we have loved helping and supporting you and Zak over the years. He's a funny, caring boy and we wouldn't wish him to be any different. I still, to this day, get people from school who I haven't spoken to in years, asking me how Zak is doing, and I love that, it makes me so proud. He is a credit to us all.'

And finally, Hope commented, 'In my opinion, family comes first and I'm glad we could help as much as we could and play a big role in Zak's life. Wouldn't have had it any other way.'

And, you've guessed it, that made me cry again.

My sister Shelley also has many fond memories of Zak growing up. 'When he packed to stay with us one

January and we took him to the Lakes, he came in jeans and teeshirt! We had to make a detour to an outdoor shop for suitable British weather clothing.'

(But at least he wasn't in his standard Cyprus dress code, consisting of just his pants!)

She added, 'One of our favourite photos is of Zak feeding his older cousin, Naomi, (who was diagnosed with CDK L5), showing the simple acceptance of disability that children have.'

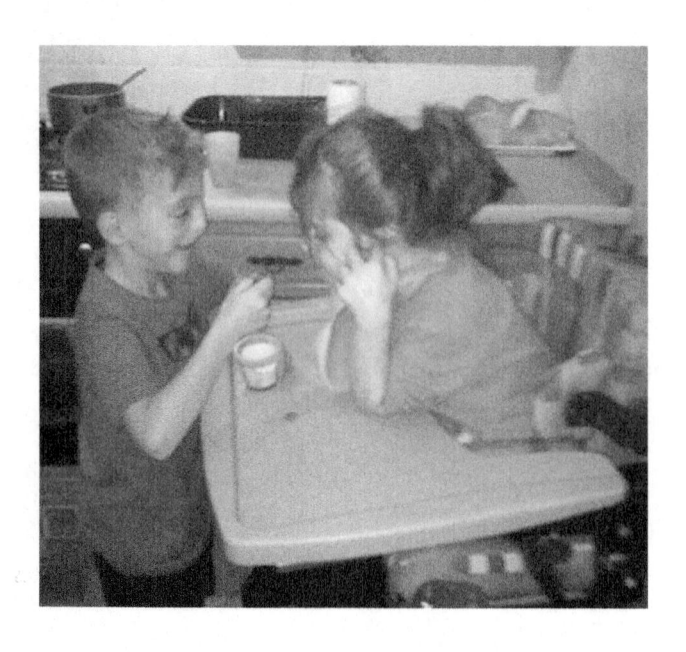

Zak feeding his cousin, Naomi

As for the other children, Jake's girls are doing well and we are in contact with them from time to time. Lucy has finished university and is now working in Newcastle while Hannah is studying at university in London.

Hannah remembers being in a shop with the family when they noticed two little boys with their mum.

'Monster,' said one of the boys.

Zak didn't respond but pulled a funny face at the boys.

'Are you okay, Zak?' Hannah asked.

'I'm fine,' he said. 'Just wanted to show them a real monster face.'

They laughed and Hannah tells me she was super proud of her little brother.

Another fond memory from Hannah is when Jake took the children to Paphos Waterpark and it rained the whole time they were there. Hannah and India hated it but Zak absolutely loved it, despite the rain and ran circles around them all.

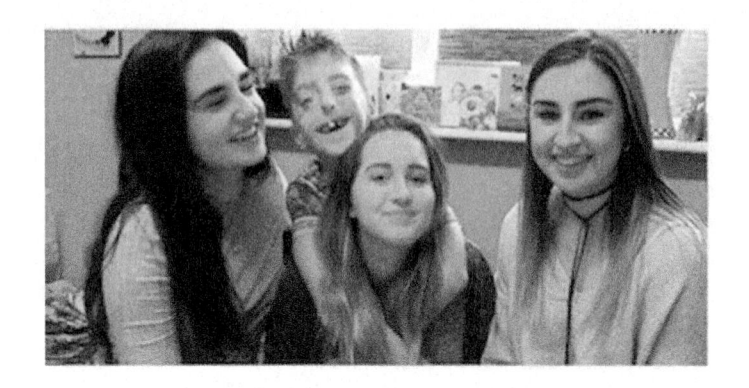

The siblings during Christmas 2017

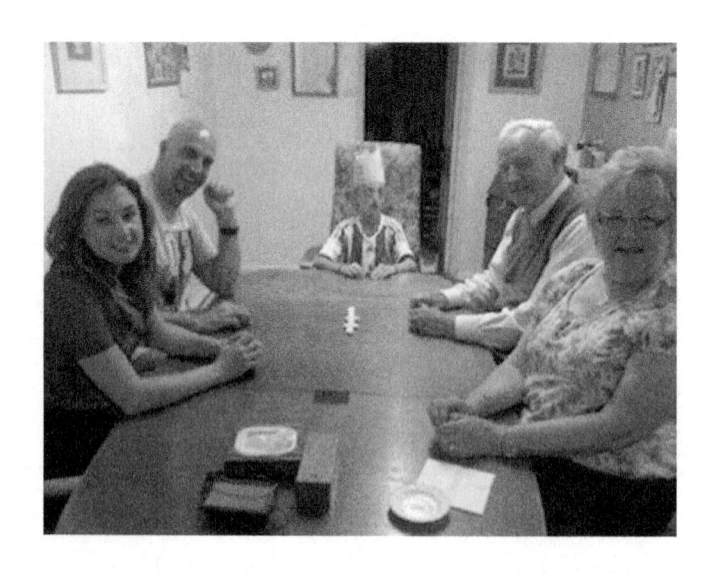

Grandmaster Zak with his father, Jake, grandparents, Dorothy and Max, and sister, Lucy

Zak has a special relationship with his grandparents and his grandmother commented, 'Zak is a special grandson and an amazing and wonderful boy. I was in Cyprus when he was born and met him at one day old – he was so tiny and precious. As I saw him each day the survival determination and strength of this baby boy was life itself. I said prayers each and every day.

'I visited Cyprus as often as I could, knowing how precious my visits were to spend time with this lovely family. When he was a little older, Zak would greet me at the airport and sit on my suitcase (on the trolley), beaming and chattering away. He would come into my bedroom early in the morning eating his breakfast or with a big smile on his face.

'It's so early, Zak,' I would say. 'Does Mummy know you're up and about?'

'But, Nanna, it's light and time to wake up.'

He was always ready to face the day with gusto.

Zak is such an independent little chap, keen to take

care of himself from a young age.

Whenever we met I would hear my favourite word; *Nanna,* said with such love and delight it made my heart swell. Granddad loved Zak's visits to York, playing games with him and taking him to visit various attractions. During a visit to his cousin's, Zak took me by the hand. 'I have something to show you,' he said, pointing to a field at the bottom of the garden. 'Look, Nanna, real cows!' He went on to tell me that he loved the UK and planned to live here one day.

'Zak has so much love and kindness for everyone and the most beautiful smile ever. We are both so proud of him and delighted to share time and life with our grandson. He makes us so happy and is always full of energy–Zak is a precious gift, who we love with all our hearts.

'My only sadness was that Joanne's Mum was unable to share in this special boy's life with us, but I believe she has been there to watch over Zak and given him the smile and strength he has. Life goes on, I am sure.'

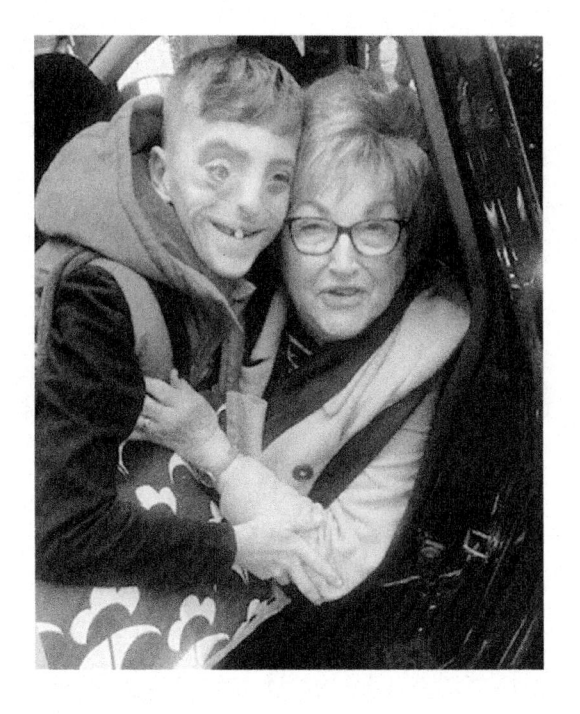

Zak with his lovely Nanna

On the wedding day of Zak's cousin Christina, Zak was in awe of how beautiful she looked and was convinced she was a real princess. He was her little shadow and followed her everywhere. Christina remains a princess to this day!

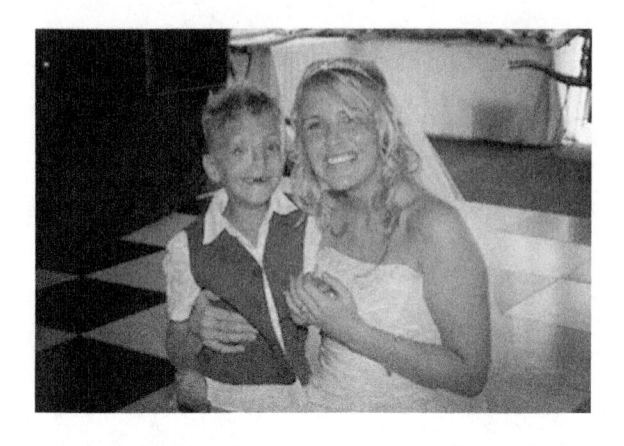

Zak and Christina

A mutual friend in Paphos put me and Helen back in touch with each other. It brought back all of the memories of our stay in Nicosia Hospital. I was messaging with Helen recently, and her words brought me to tears, 'Meeting Zak enabled David to get first-hand experience of seeing a child with facial differences, and to ask questions. He now embraces disabilities, be they mental or physical, and shows compassion. There is a girl we know who is severely mentally handicapped who goes giddy when she sees David and instead of walking AWAY he takes time to say hello and high-five her. I put that down to speaking honestly to him about Zak. I will always remember his happy face when watching Zak's video of his Floss Dance.'

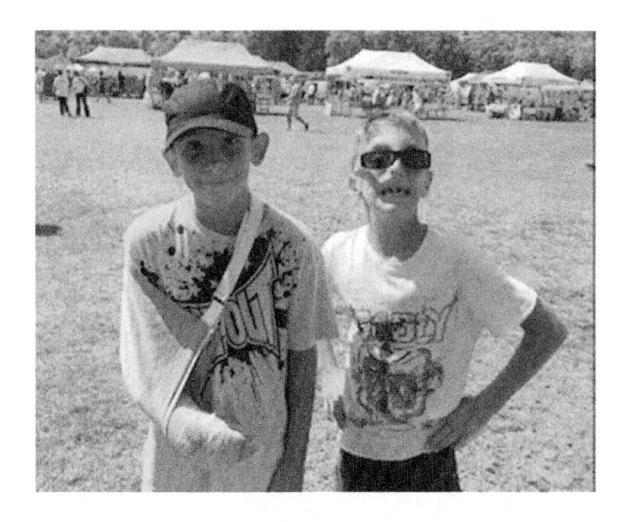

Zak and David meet for the first time since being premature babies together

A little while ago I decided to embark on a fitness regime and have run in a number of races. Not wanting to be left out, Zak decided to join me and here he is posing before his first 5k race in Larnaca last year. Debbi, my personal trainer, did his pre-run warm-up exercises with him. It was a proud mummy moment when he finished in 38 minutes and hadn't even trained for the event!

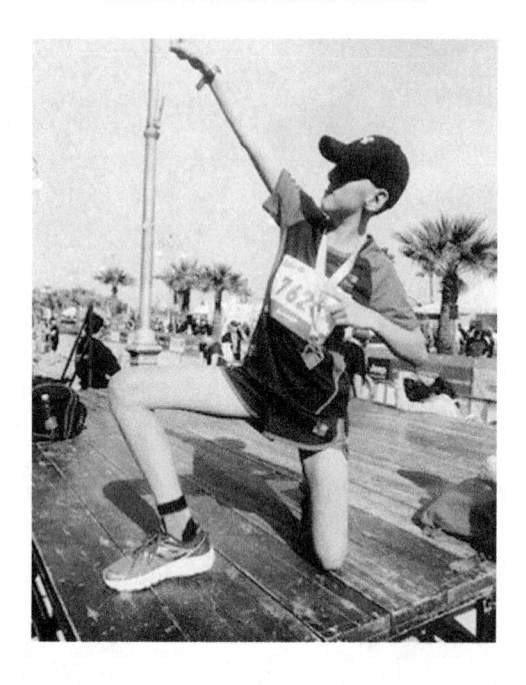

Zak's impersonation of that very famous sportsman

As for me, I spent most of Zak's formative years bringing up my children on my own, and although it's been tough, it has also been very satisfying. I'm blessed with some wonderful friends (cheesy I know, but it's true!) who have been and continue to be very supportive. Jake works in another country and Zak recently spent his first holiday there with his dad and had a fab time.

I'm extremely proud of my wonderful daughter,

India, who is an intelligent, caring, and happy young woman, and of my miracle boy who is kind, considerate, and charismatic. Both are a joy to be around.

Whatever the future holds, my kids are my world. I consider myself lucky to be able to share my life with two such special people; one who has managed to survive everything against all the odds, and made us all appreciate what is really important in this life.

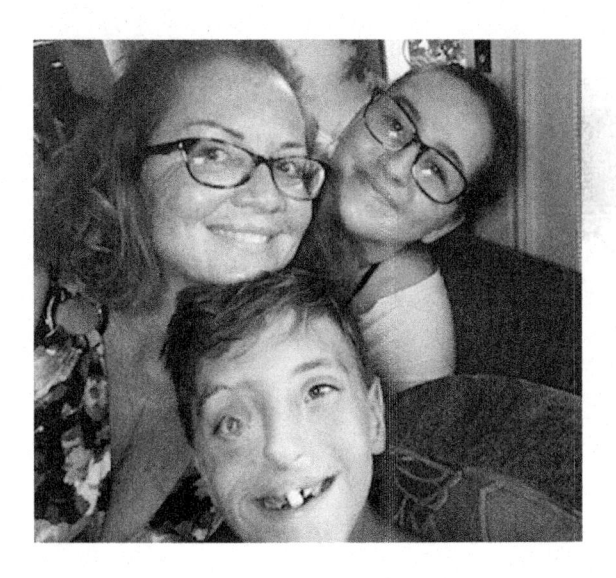

My kids, my life, my world

From Zak

When we asked Zak if he wanted to add anything to this book he said, 'No matter what they say I will always slay them from my mind and with all the courage I gain from my Mummy she will never fade away from my side.'

That made me cry, again – Jo.

He also added, 'Don't be worried, don't be shy, and even though people may say things, they are ignorant and they don't know what's inside of you. Be proud of your achievements. Don't feel down about how you look, be proud of your cleft. Always remember your family and friends will be by your side.'

My Boy Wonder

Born far too soon, my baby boy
He filled my heart with love and joy.
They said he wouldn't last a day.
The vicar came and we all prayed.
My Boy Wonder.

The months ahead were touch and go,
His progress was so very slow.
I held him in the dark of night,
Made deals with God he'd be all right.
My Boy Wonder.

The dream team medics had a plan,
My baby went through tests and scans.
They'd build his face and make him well,
Would this work out? Just time would tell.
My Boy Wonder.

The operations soon begun,
He was so brave, my lovely son.
And when some people stopped to stare
They had to deal with Mama Bear!
My Boy Wonder.

He smiles a lot and is so kind,
But not afraid to speak his mind.
He helps those who are weak or frail,
When Zak's around, the bullies fail.
My Boy Wonder.

He's thirteen now, the years have flown,
And how my little boy has grown.
More ops and grafts are on the cards,
And life is good, though sometimes hard.
My Boy Wonder.

I see my brave and cherished son,
And marvel at how well he's done.
My heart swells up with love and pride,
This life has dealt us quite a ride.
My Boy Wonder.

No matter what our future plan,
As Zak grows up from boy to man.
I see him through a mummy's eyes,
And this won't come as a surprise...
He'll always be My Boy Wonder.

(by Deb McEwan – Copyright 2019)

Final Thoughts from Jo

Thank you, first of all, to Zak's father, Jake, for the wonderful boy we made together. To my fabulous daughter, India (a second mum to Zak as she's grown up), and to his two other big sisters who also love him unconditionally. To all the medical professionals, (especially those already mentioned in this book) who have looked after Zak and my family since he came into this world. Special thanks to the Edwards' (thanks Hope and Robyn for willingly giving up your bedrooms every time we visited) and Ashton families AKA my sisters and their families. To Ashra, who has been with us since before Zak was born and has treated my children like her own - Zak has always been able to wrap Ashra around his little finger! To my close friends (Liz, Gina, Elena, Lilli, and Deb, to name but a few) who, over the years, have always been there for me. To Jake's family who have continually kept in touch and supported us, especially Dorothy and Max, Julie, and Christina. Thanks, too, to our fabulous editor, Jill Turner, for helping to make this book the best that it can be, and for our awesome elite team of advanced readers (Julie, Trudy, Su, Tina, Debbie, Helen, Libby, James, Lou, and Maddie) – you rock!

Thank you for purchasing this book. We hope you enjoyed it (now that you know there's a happy ending) and would love it if you shared your thoughts and wrote a review.

If you'd like to know more about Changing Faces – the charity for people with visual facial differences - you can visit their Facebook page here.
https://www.facebook.com/ChangingFacesUK/

To contact me, use this link,
https://www.facebook.com/joanne.lythgoe or to contact Deb or discover more about her fiction books check out the following links:
https://www.facebook.com/DebMcEwansbooksandblogs/?ref=bookmarks
or
https://www.debmcewansbooksandblogs.com

If you'd like to follow the Cleft Lip and Palate Association (CLAPA), their Facebook page is here
https://www.facebook.com/groups/199800453464048/

You might also like to know

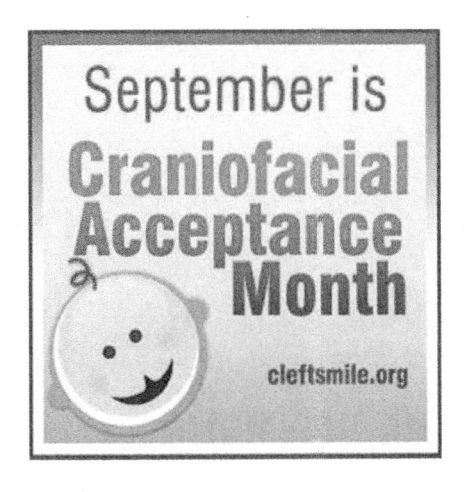

September is Craniofacial Acceptance Month

cleftsmile.org

Printed in Great Britain
by Amazon